13.00 +x

About the Author and the Book

Humans are the only species that regularly eat what is bad for them and makes them sick. In contrast, wild animals are selective in what they eat and do not suffer from the chronic diseases and cancers suffered by humans, pets and zoo animals raised on processed food. Even wild bears with all that body fat live healthy lives without any diabetes medication! Today, humans with access to processed food and expensive medicines live about 25% of their lives with pain, disease and declining energy (vitality). In the US, we spend 20-25% of our GDP on treating the sick.

Good food is essential for nourishing our *guts,* otherwise known as our "second brain" because they are innervated by the second largest neural network in the body (after our brain). Our intestines also host the largest bacterial colony in the body, which produce modulators of our immune system, mood, digestion and metabolism. Yet, much of the food we eat today ravages our digestive tract instead of nourishing it because food is now a profitable *commodity* carefully designed, denatured and marketed to maximize corporate profits and not its metabolic contribution to our body.

Ray Armat, Ph.D., a graduate of University of Michigan and Case Western Reserve University, is a polymath, food packaging expert and former NASA grantee who shares with us his own unbiased research about food metabolism. As a farmer scientist, he offers simple dietary principles and rules of thumb for eating well, plus little-disclosed facts about eggs, dairy, fruits, meat, gluten and detox protocols. Visit RayArmat.com for his other writin

The Right Way to Eat

A Handbook About Wholesome Food

Ray Armat, Ph.D.

The Right Way to Eat
A Handbook About Wholesome Food

First published Newport, Pennsylvania in the United States of America by Applied Analytic Research Inc.

ISBN 979-8-9859694-7-4 (paperback)

Printed in the United States of America
First Edition 2024

Cover Design by CookieDoh Studios LLC

Dedicated

To readers like you who have the courage to be vulnerable, the humility to self-reflect, and the wisdom to trust your time to a non-famous thinker.

And

To my family who taught me patience and contentment with simple joys in life: Nature, faith, books, farming, music (banjo, violin), love, and best home-made food!

Warning:

I have been told my content evokes a strong response from some interest groups, which would try to limit my reach. If you are looking for a book from yet another "attention merchant" who confirms your biases, this book may not be for you! I have spared myself no pains to be scientifically objective and respectful of all views and humans. Yet being guided just by my God-given conscience, not by book sales, fame, politics, narratives or dogmas, I won't "sugar coat" my observations.

Table of Contents

1
What does Health Mean?

Did you know that long ago, there was only one species on this planet fit enough to outlast gazelles in long chases and hunt them? "Persistence hunting" took place during the hottest time of the day and involved chasing a fat-running animal like a gazelle for hours until it was outrun to exhaustion and captured. But who could outlast a gazelle? The answer is our distant ancestors and early humans.

Humans *used to be* among the best "endurance runners" on this planet, which had its adaptive advantages because before farming or domestication of hound dogs, "persistence hunting" was an efficient form of securing food by some humans. If we define *health* as *endurance,* humans used to be a healthy species.

Although biologists attribute human endurance to our ability to sweat and cool down in warmer weather, our ancestors had superb endurance even in colder months and when clothed and not sweating. For example, consider Edward Marshall, one of the fastest runners in the American colony of Pennsylvania, commissioned by the Penn family during *The Walking Purchase of Pennsylvania* in 1737 to resolve a land border dispute with the native American Lenape tribe. Marshall walked and ran for 1.5 days to cover a distance of 70 miles, which gave the colonists a land area roughly 1.2 million acres – 70 miles by 70 miles or 4900 square miles. Edward Marshall took no medications or performance-enhancing drugs and had no access to fancy gyms. He ate little but *good natural unprocessed* food. Imagine walking non-stop for a day and a half over rugged hills, mountains, thick old-growth forests, rivers and valleys of Northeast Pennsylvania. Marshall carried a hatchet and threw it from one hand to the other as he walked to balance his gait, and also used it to cut away brushes and branches in his way.

A century later, young poor boys and orphans who led the mules towing cargo boats along the towpaths of water canals in Pennsylvania, walked for six hours straight in all sorts of weather on one *good* meal a day.

There is no doubt that it was the *right type of food* our ancestors ate that made them resilient. Even today, people aged 90 years or older whose formative years in childhood were before World War II and the era of industrial denatured processed food, often seem more resilient and lively than younger people of newer generations. My own father who grew up impoverished before World War II on a diet of whole grains (barley bread), potato, herbs, walnuts, and fruits – fresh and dried like raisins – worked long hours as an old-fashioned carpenter without any power tools like drills and saws, and kept his vigor and vitality until he immigrated to America around the age of 65 and started eating 'SAD' (Standard American Diet). He was soon put on medications until he died at the age of 86.

Today, most humans cannot even walk a few miles let alone run and outlast a gazelle for eight hours, or clear a 70-mile rugged path in a thick forest within a day with a hatchet, or cut wood and lumber for hours with hand saws. Our ancestors were usually skinnier but more virile and vital than us. The word *vitality* comes from the Latin word *vita*, which means "life."

Life and health are indeed both linked to *energy*. In my first book, I quoted Nobel Laureate Albert Szent-Györgyi, the distinguished biochemist who isolated vitamin C and identified the metabolic process in living cells (the Krebs cycle) from his book *The Living State with Observations on Cancer*:

"*As shown so delightfully by Schrodinger in his little book 'What is Life?', the main characteristic of life is that it tends to decrease its entropy. It also tends to increase its free energy.*"

Thermodynamically, "free energy" is the maximum energy our body (or any system) has available for *physical* (motion-related) work[1]. By this definition, many lethargic or fatigued humans today with low energy levels are *partially alive* and suffer from poor *vitality* and metabolism (the conversion of food to energy).

Modern humans have developed sophisticated tools and foods to stay "healthy" without even pondering the meaning of "health."[2] Many people equate health with longevity and just living longer even with pain, low energy and metabolic diseases like diabetes or cancer!

Brilliant scientists like Szent-Györgyi have noticed that cancer is caused by a chaotic metabolism and loss of free energy in humans, which I also blame for *social* chaos and disorder. All living organisms are intelligently designed to self-heal and share energy and life with each other. In other words, we get our energy from eating vegetables, grains or meat, which are all living organisms. Vegetables continue breathing and ripening even after being cut. If we eat sick or partially-alive food (with low "free energy"), we can expect to be sick and partially-alive. Most food we consume today is of low quality of energy and vitality.

If you believe in the soul or God, our *spiritual energy* also depends on a wholesome body. The Bible refers to the human body as "The Temple of the Holy Spirit," which we cannot defile or abuse. Our food becomes our body's building blocks. Would you live in a house built with rotten lumber, leaky pipes and frayed wires? Our bodies age and fall apart further each time we feed them low-quality food. Our spiritual energy dwindles each time we use cheap building blocks for *The Temple.*

The quality of the food we eat also directly affects the quality of our sleep, which is the single most important

---

[1] I have explained the concept of "Gibbs free energy" in my first book

[2] A good book on the topic is "Mirage of Health" by René Dubos

part of our life for proper healing, mental health, and recharging spiritual and physical "batteries."

If you want evidence of the importance of food quality on the *vitality* of a living organism, you need to look no further than in zoos. Studies have shown that zoo animals are sicker or smaller than wild animals partly because of the denatured diet in captivity. For example, research by Adam Hartstone-Rose shows that *male* lions and tigers in captivity fed with heavily processed diets were comparable in size and strength to *females in the wild* and smaller than their wild male counterparts. Zoo animals also suffer from a variety of health issues including gut issues and poor dental health, also impacting the humans running these zoos! This can be partly caused by denatured zoo diets which, according to the Association of Zoos and Aquariums, cannot have any bones, cartilage, organs, skin or connective tissues. *Denatured* food makes *any* organism *denatured* and sick.

In fact, humans are probably the only species who are not selective or picky about what they eat. Multiple observational studies, including one by Madeleine Hansell, point out that most animals in the wild are highly selective feeders and display preferences for certain types of plants or plant parts. They carefully select their food based on the nutritional and/or toxic content of the source and what is *seasonally* available. Many animals are known to avoid food containing antinutrients like alkaloids, phenolics or tannins that are toxic or inhibit the digestion of proteins and starch.

Evidence shows that unlike pets raised by humans on processed food and suffering from diabetes, blood pressure and cancer, wild or free-ranging animals which selectively feed on their preferred (natural) diet do not suffer from chronic diseases. Even bears with all that body fat live long and healthy lives - unless humans hunt them, destroy their natural habitat, or kill them in road accidents – without any insulin shots or diabetes medicine. Without relying on good food for vitality and energy, wild animals like squirrels and rabbits could not feed or breed so vigorously. In my first book, to show my readers how metabolically inefficient humans are, I calculated the flight fuel (caloric) efficiency of some migratory birds like blackpoll warblers as equivalent to about 720,000 miles per gallon (in human terms)! These birds just rely on metabolizing the good natural food they consume, without borrowing from fossil or landlocked fuels, like humans do.

The life of wild animals, if not shortened abruptly by a predator, naturally ends following a short period of lethargy, immobility and metabolic exhaustion. For free-ranging pasture-raised chickens, this morbidity period is usually less than two days, which would be equivalent to a couple weeks of human lifespan. Contrast that with the 20-30 years of declining energy, health and vitality experienced in later life by humans today with access to all kinds of processed food and expensive medicines. By many accounts, the *health span* of people in industrial countries is 20-30 years shorter than their *lifespan.*, which means, on average, people live 25% of their lives unhealthy and in various forms of pain and imbalance. Actually, in the United States, medical and health-care (actually, 'sick-care') spending is about 20-25% of our GDP – Gross Domestic Product. So once you exclude the non-productive age groups, our adult population indeed spends about 25% of its working hours paying for the country's morbidity-related medical bills. I believe with healthy food (not denatured) and lifestyles, people could work less, have more joy and vitality (energy), and not burden the fiscal budgets for medical and sick-care systems.

I have discovered a lot of evidence about the long *health spans* of ancient people eating natural food. For example, the first century Jewish historian Joseph[redacted]e
us

mentions in *Jewish Wars, Book II. Chapter 8* that many members of the pacifist Essene community lived "*more than a hundred years because of the simplicity of their diet and the regular course of life they observe.*" There is evidence to indicate that Jesus and John the Baptist were close to this ancient Jewish sect, which followed a diet of fresh fruit, vegetables, whole grains (barley and wheat), almonds, milk and honey, figs or dates.

I have also seen a reference in *Golestan* (which means "The Flower Garden"), the 13th century wisdom book by Persian poet *Saadi* to his personal visitation to a 150-year-old man who was fearful of dying.

Even if you don't believe the Biblical stories about the long lives of pre-flood prophets like Noah, Abraham and Methuselah, there are a lot of other references to long-living healthy humans before the industrial and digital age. In a research article published on BBC, Amanda Ruggeri demonstrates that life expectancy in ancient Rome and in the Victorian period was not markedly different from what it is today. In fact, excluding the large number of people who died in infancy, in wars or in polluted cities, life spans were probably higher in ancient times than what they are today with all our access to cheap and abundant food.

As I will explain in this book, the lower prices and larger quantities of mass-produced food in the industrial age are made possible by *denaturing* pure food sources and sacrificing their quality and bioavailability. I have designed and invented several food packaging concepts in the past. In the next few chapters I will share with you some of the ways modern food is denatured and adulterated. As a result of these drastic changes in recent years, there have been endless debates about foods that are most natural and beneficial for our health. In search of an answer, about one hundred years ago, Dr. Weston Price, a prominent dentist from Cleveland, Ohio, decided to travel around the world to study isolated human groups who still had perfectly healthy teeth, balanced disease-free bodies and emotionally stable demeanors. After analyzing the food used by these indigenous peoples, Price concluded that the best diet for humans is one rich in minerals (calcium, magnesium, potassium, etc.) and fat-soluble vitamins A, D, E and K found in nutrient-dense whole foods, including vegetables and raw animal products like unpasteurized milk, eggs and organ meat.

Although some of these findings have been controversial, there is indisputable evidence that shows when migrant humans change their diet from traditional natural foods to modern processed foods, diseases and morbidity follow. I already mentioned the story of my own father. He doesn't seem to be an exception. According to an article by Sabrina Tavernise in the NY Times, mortality data on immigrants shows that the longer they live in the US, the worse their rates of heart disease, high blood pressure and diabetes.

About 50% of all Americans are now either diabetic or pre-diabatic (fasting glucose of 100 or higher) which is unprecedented in history and in nature when compared to a natural (healthy) incidence rate of zero, seen in the wild or among our ancestors just some 80 years ago. Yet, there seems to be no resolve in educating people about the dietary roots of this health crisis. There is a lot of money to be made in patching up the largest single market segment in America!

The American Diabetes Association, the main organization that directs scientific policies and academic research to identify the root causes of this crisis, is mainly funded by the pharmaceutical companies that manufacture weight loss, diabetes and blood sugar regulator drugs and monitoring devices! And by pharmacy chains like CVS. The motto for another major Diabetes foundation is now "Living with Diabetes" instead of preventing it! Researchers Daniel Aaron and Michael Siegel documented that companies making sugary food and beverages heavily sponsor national health and medical organizations to fund research that underplays the role of sugary and processed food in diseases such as heart disease or diabetes, while concurrently lobbying against any public health bill intended to improve nutrition.

It is scientifically certain that low-quality and denatured foods are directly responsible for ravaging our metabolism and for creating the current chronic disease crisis. Even when it comes to dreaded infectious diseases (like COVID-19), many people do not realize that the progression from *infection* to *disease* requires a *dysfunctional metabolism* and immune system. In the words of renowned microbiologist René Dubos:

"*It is barely recognized, but nevertheless true, that animals and plants, as well as men, can live peacefully with their most notorious microbial enemies .. millions of young people become infected by polio viruses, yet suffer no harm.. infection can occur without producing disease.*"

So if we define "health" as a healthy *metabolism*, which also drives our *vitality*, healthy food is any food which does not disrupt our *natural metabolic balance.*

As part of the research for my first two books and for the best dietary guidelines for my own family, I have been studying the impact of food ingredients on our *metabolic health* and energy levels. There are numerous books and videos about diet and health with conflicting advice, causing frustration in people. My research shows that there are no one-size-fits-all universal miracle diets because everyone's metabolic needs and immune system is unique. This book is not intended to substitute medical advice or promote any sponsored product. Guided by my conscience, and not book sales or politics, I share simple guidelines and rules of thumb that anyone can use to make wise food choices. I have used *italics*, **bold** or underlined for key concepts.

Before we start exploring food, I would like to point out the worldwide epidemics of constipation, sleep, smell and sexual disorders, which I call the 4 S's of dysfunction in modern life: Stool, Sleep, Smelling and Sexual disorders. In my first two books, I have shown the connection between these disorders and our denatured lifestyles and diets. According to research by Sorangel Diaz, constipation is now reported in about 30% of children and 40% of adults over 65. Worldwide, constipation rates in many countries now approach 50% and are matched by incidence rates of sleep, smell and sexual dysfunction. Research by Henry Duboc links digestive disorders like constipation and irritable bowel syndrome to maladjusted (chaotic) circadian rhythms of body functions like sleep. This is a short excerpt from my recent book *The Rogue Brain*:

"*We are also the only species that does not know what's best for us to eat, drink, watch, etc. ... Years of research, debate and schooling has not brought us into agreement about the dietary or lifestyle roots of our diseases. While trying to control the universe, we are still ignorant about how our body, mind and soul (spirit) connect with each other. As modern humans are getting closer to conquering Mars, they have a long way to figuring out how to control their gut issues and constipation at home.*"

Today, food, medicine and supplements are big *global* (non-local) profitable businesses. There is a lot of *misinformation* and conflicts of interest out there. Major food businesses own divisions that make cigarettes and alcohol or support weight loss medications while selling foods that induce weight gain! The maker of herbicides used on our grains, suspected to cause non-Hodgkin's lymphoma (cancer), also makes money by developing anti-cancer drugs! It is essential for all of us to be wise and educated about our nourishment.

Chapter 1: The Food's Journey Inside Our Body

Every system in the universe, including our body and the food we eat, has some mass, momentum (movement force) and energy, which changes its form over time. As taught to scientists and chemical engineers in universities, every process in the world involves exchanges and transfers of mass, momentum and/or energy. For example, when we cook potatoes in boiling water, we are transferring the energy reserves of the fuel on fire to the metal pot which, being a good conductor of heat, will transfer most of that energy to the water (and some of that to the air around it). Water will in turn transfer some of that energy to the potatoes, but also uses some energy to heat itself up, mobilize its molecules, break their bonds, and ultimately reach its boiling point. The reason boiling is such a great way to transfer heat to and from fluids is the enormous energy needed to move fluid molecules from liquid to a vapor state – during boiling or evaporation. That is why steam burns our skin worse than hot water does. The immense energy absorbed by the boiling water ends up with the steam and with the potato. If the pot has a lid, most of that steam stays in and will build pressure (another form of energy, transferred to the headspace of the pot) and give some back to the potato again. All of that heat transferred to the potato causes its cell membranes and starch molecules – *polysaccharides*, which means "many sugar molecules," are long chains of glucose molecules chemically bonded together – to break down and allow some water in. In time, this moisture will turn into steam, expand, and cause the starch grains to rupture further to starch granules or smaller molecules – like *monosaccharides*, meaning "one sugar molecule" – which are easier for our body to digest. The swelling and bursting of starch molecules begin at 137–150 °F (58–66 °C) and speed up at boiling point near 212 °F.

Let's go deeper with our mass and energy transfer analysis. The energy of the fire itself comes from the chemical bonds in the carbon-based "fuel" like wood or propane, which release their bonding energy by reacting with oxygen and generating heat (flame), carbon dioxide and water. So it's a mass and energy exchange at the same time. The water and carbon dioxide molecules are released by the fire as you are cooking and carry some energy away into your kitchen's airspace. The energy in the fuel's chemical bonds were packed there years ago, when smaller carbon-based molecules were ordered, organized, packed and compacted by an external energy source like sunlight. So, the wood in a tree, the same as the starch molecules in the potato, are both organized long-chain molecules (polymers) which are basically nature's tools to condense, store (like a battery) and transfer "energy" packets of the abundant sunlight on our planet. The wood is broken down during combustion to release the stored energy to the potato, which uses that energy to break down its starch into molecules small enough for human digestion. Many energy sources in nature, like tubers and roots consumed heavily by our early ancestors, needed a lot of chewing energy to break them down into smaller digestible molecules. Inventions like fire or fermentation – discussed in a later chapter – gave our ancestors an advantage over animals such as wild chimps, which spend hours a day chewing their fibrous diet. Wasting less of our own energy on breaking down our food, we have more calories available for our physical and brain growth.

The powerful and energy-hungry human brains have invented easy to digest, cheap and concentrated – in other words, *denatured* – energy sources like pure sugar and finely ground flour/grains. These easy fuels do not even require long baking, fermentation or even chewing to release their stored energy. As I explained in my book

The Rogue Brain, nothing pleases the modern human brain more than convenience, speed, and scale (quantity). Denatured non-fresh sources of calories which are highly-processed and chemically-preserved are convenient, cheap and abundant (scalable). They typically have a long shelf-life in the stores and kitchens, and can be conveniently purchased and consumed without a lot of physical work. Farming (for fresh fruits, vegetables and grains), hunting or fishing (for fresh meat), peeling, boiling, fermenting, grinding, or even chewing all required physical work. Contrast that with the effortless consumption of soft, low-fiber processed foods. Today, few households in the industrialized world cook their meals regularly using fresh and non-concentrated, non-processed raw ingredients. Even fewer people fish, farm or hunt their own food. As a result, almost nothing is fresh, local, baked or cooked. We will explore why this is disastrous for our health, and our income too.

Since our bodies constantly break down mass to release energy stored in that mass, we are part of the energy transfer chain on this planet that includes the potato, the water in the pot, the wood burned to boil the water, as well as the living soil (not chemically-treated) that nourished the tree (fuel) and the potato (food). It is all about transfer of mass and energy in nature to sustain life. And life is the only force in nature that imposes order over chaos, supports our movements and increases our free energy – a thermodynamic concept explained in my previous books. Good food produces the life force (vitality) needed for cellular level order, balance and movement. Bad food creates imbalance, cellular disorders as seen in cancer, and low free energy and movement. In fact, upon death, cells become disordered and we become immobile. Many humans today, kept alive by expensive medical interventions, may not be dead but lack vitality and live a life of disease, cellular disorder and immobility due in part to their food choices and habits.

Life relies on the energy transfer between living organisms, and since our digestion process is part of that supply and transfer chain, the less *denatured* our food is, the more we are in harmony with our food sources and their natural state of balance.

The Digestion Process

We learned that in baking or boiling potatoes, we borrow outside energy sources to break down some of the long carbon chains into simpler sugars (saccharides or glucose) digestible by our digestive tract. But what happens to these saccharides when we eat that boiled potato? Well, a single glucose molecule still has several chemical bonds with a lot of energy to be released inside our body. Basically, the process of releasing the energy stored in glucose requires oxidation and is chemically very similar to releasing the energy stored in other carbohydrates (like wood) or hydrocarbons (propane or oil) by oxidation (burning). The burning of glucose as fuel happens inside our cells – in an organelle called mitochondria – with the help of oxygen supplied by our blood. Oxygen is transferred from our lungs to our cells by hemoglobins and red blood cells, which act like delivery boats. These hemoglobins and red blood cells also carry the combustion product of carbon dioxide back to our lungs, which is then released there as we exhale.

However, even baked potatoes with plenty of bioavailable glucose need to be first processed and vetted by our body before it's allowed to reach our cells and release its energy for our movement and vitality.

From the minute we start chewing our food, our intelligent sensors in the mouth, tongue, and along the digestive tract (esophagus, stomach, small and large intestines) start assessing and metabolizing the food to benefit us. For example, when we eat and chew leafy green vegetables like lettuce, our body senses molecules called nitrates and unleashes our mouth bacteria[3] to break the nitrates down to nitric oxide. This nitric oxide not only reduces oral acidity and prevents the growth of harmful bacteria that can cause gum disease and tooth decay, it also dilates our blood vessels and help decrease our blood pressure[4] when it reaches our gut and is absorbed in the bloodstream.

Whether it's lettuce or baked potato, chewing well – say at least 20 times – and mixing the food with our mouth's good bacteria and enzymes – makes the job of our stomach acid easier in breaking down the food to its digestible components and building blocks.

The main components and types of building blocks in food, and what each does for our body, are outlined in the next chapter.

Depending on how well we have chewed the food, how much we have eaten, and how difficult the food is to break down, the food can typically spend 2-4 hours in our stomach. During this period, there is a lot of blood flow to the stomach to support its churning action and acidification to break down food. Foods high in fat and protein, and low in carbohydrates, water, and acid content typically stay longer in the stomach. This is why some people feel cold or sleepy after eating heavy meals. It is not good to lay down during this time or do any strenuous activity. It is also not good to be stressed over work or life projects, argue with people, rush eating, or engage in any other activity that triggers our brain's stress response and hormones adrenaline and cortisol, which

---

[3] Antiseptic mouthwashes may temporarily mask odors, but they can also kill some of the most beneficial bacteria and biosensors in our mouth

[4] Too much nitrate, found in non-organic lettuce grown with synthetic ammonium nitrate fertilizers, could form N-nitrosamines in the body, which is linked to cancer in humans.

paralyze our digestive functions. It is best to enjoy food slowly and calmly in a peaceful setting preferably away from digital media (TV, phones) and all other stressors of life and work, and in the company of nature or people you trust or enjoy. Standing up or walking slowly after eating is OK and helpful. Before each meal, pausing, praying for grace or at least taking several deep breaths will slow down our unruly brain and make us more grateful and attentive to the life-giving experience of eating.

Chewing the food thoroughly and patiently, and trying to savor every hint of aroma and flavor in each bite of good food, will help us digest the food and keep our body vital and our senses sharp. Cheap poor quality food may look nice but often has no *natural* aroma or flavor so we often just devour and swallow it instead of savoring the aroma in every bite we chew. Good food needs few if any seasonings and definitely no artificial additives, preservatives or colors. Good food is naturally packed with its own aroma and flavors that attract our senses. Once we train our senses to savor good food, we will no longer be attracted to bad food. For example, once you savor the aroma and flavor of a locally-grown and seasonal chemical-free tomato (the type we grow on our farm), which is vine-ripened and hand cultivated, you will no longer be inclined to waste your money on conventional (sprayed) flavorless pricey tomatoes from mechanized farms. Let's get back to the digestion process.

The partially-digested paste expelled by the stomach into the duodenum (opening of the small intestine) is called chyme or chymus. Depending on what our body senses in the chyme, it will release additional hormones and digestive juices to metabolize it. For example, the brain signals an organ called pancreas, sitting right under the stomach, to release digestive juices (called pancreatic enzymes) into the upper part of our small intestine to help break down foods further. The body monitors the levels of sugars and fats released into the bloodstream during this process. When blood sugar levels are too high, the pancreas releases a hormone called insulin into the bloodstream to activate all our cells to use up glucose and "burn" it or "bury" it as fat stores. When blood sugar levels are too low, or fat or amino acids (proteins) levels are too high, the pancreas releases a hormone called glucagon into the bloodstream, which signals our body (cells) to "break down" fat and other energy reserves into sugar and release it into the blood (you can find more details in a paper by Jiudan Zhang). Many of our organs like kidneys, liver, brain, intestines, heart and fat cells work together and sense these signaling metabolic hormones in the bloodstream to optimize our digestion and metabolism. Our body is an intelligent biochemical factory that constantly Builds, Buries, Breaks down or Burns molecules, which I call the 4B's of metabolism. Our liver alone, for example, performs over 500 vital functions and molecular conversions depending on the type of food we eat and molecules we release into our bloodstream every day.

Each time we overload and stress our digestive system with *denatured* or *unnaturally-processed* food, we throw off our hormonal balance (insulin, glucagon, etc.) and functionality of our organs – like liver – and the whole body. For example, overeating processed foods containing denatured forms of glucose such as pure sugar or high fructose corn syrup overloads our pancreas and insulin systems, and can lead to insulin-resistance (diabetes) or pancreatic cancer.

A lot of times, our stationary body does not even need all the food and excess calories imposed on it by our anxious brain that demands sugary food and excess calories to appease itself in times of *psychological* stress. My book *The Rogue Brain* explains how most of our digestive problems and metabolic diseases are rooted in our unruly brains, and how rebuilding (detoxifying) the body with good food can help us recondition our brains to kick their junk food addiction and other bad habits.

Our body is intelligent enough to metabolize the food we eat and convert it to most vitamins and all the hormones (signaling molecules) it needs with cues and help by natural sunlight in how much of each hormone to make or release in the body. In fact, prior to the invention of electric light and digital distractors our ancestors only ate and slept in harmony with natural daily cycles and circadian rhythms. The body of natural humans, like most mammals, got their cues from early morning and seasonal sunlight in making metabolic hormones and biochemicals such as dopamine (motivating us to feed and breed), cortisol and adrenaline (energizing us to focus and handle stress), and testosterone or estrogens (reproductive hormones).

We now know that our skin cells contain the entire biochemical apparatus necessary to be activated by the ultraviolet (UV) radiation in sunlight, and vitamins A, B, C, D, E, and Zinc to convert cholesterol molecules into hormones like cortisol, testosterone, progesterone, estrogens and aldosterone – the antidiuretic hormone retaining sodium and water for adequate blood pressure. Any malfunction in this system, with bad food and lifestyle, leads to all sorts of inflammatory disorders and autoimmune diseases, according to research by Andrzej Slominski and others. In simple terms, all our body needs for proper functioning, energy metabolism and hormonal balance is good food and sleep, low psychological stress and timely exposure to sunlight. This is a fact our schools and doctors need to share with countless humans plagued by fatigue or burnout, anxiety, depression or addiction, constipation, sleep and sexual disorders.

Because cholesterol is so important in producing several hormones, particularly male (testosterone) and female (progesterone and estrogens) sex hormones, diets that are too low in fat or fibers (which our gut bacteria can convert to small fat molecules) can be problematic. This is probably why some super skinny women or men may struggle with fertility.

Besides regulating our sex hormones, fat tissues in our body perform other important metabolic functions such as communicating to our brain the state of our fat (energy) reserves. For example, fat tissues host a hormone called Leptin, which is a messenger molecule sent to our brain to indicate fullness, adequate energy reserve, satiety, and lack of hunger. This is so the brain can order the body to stop eating and increase its base metabolic rate to burn some calories, an action mediated by the thyroid hormone. As I explained in my previous book, the high-maintenance modern human brain, driven in times of pain or stress by pleasure seeking, often ignores Leptin signals and keeps asking the body to binge on caloric food like ice cream, sugary desserts and alcohol until the brain feels "high" enough to handle its state of psychological – not physical – stress. This type of hunger and craving is psychological and not real (limbic).

If we eat when we are not truly hungry, the body will accumulate more fat cells and Leptin, and increase its base metabolism through several functions, such as sweating or staying awake. If this keeps happening in response to cravings of a chronically-stressed brain, the brain will become Leptin-resistant and the body will become insulin-resistant (diabetic).

So it's crucial for all of us to condition ourselves to listen to our body for signs of *real hunger* which include feeling a bit weak and craving for food in our entire body, particularly in our gut and our mouth, and not psychological or *stress-induced hunger*, which our brain imposes on us as a means to prevent depression.

When and What to Eat?

So far, I have discussed how our body can regulate its metabolic needs if we eat good food in proper time windows. But what are these foods and time windows? As already discussed, in nature, food consumption like all other functions follows a circadian and seasonal pattern. Our chickens, for example, start eating soon after sunlight. They peck more on worms and grass and go broody (ready for new baby chicks) in the spring and summer months. It is also important for humans to follow natural circadian rhythms in eating and sleeping to the extent possible. Artificial lights, digital devices, and psychological stressors throw off these natural rhythms which are linked to our hormonal health and balance. New research shows flat circadian profiles of hormones like cortisol are closely associated with depression. In other words, if our eating and energy metabolism habits are out-of-sync with nature, we are prone to be energetically exhausted and depressed.

It is important to eat when we feel *real hunger* and away from psychological, work or digital stressors, and stop eating when we are fairly full (not overflowing!). If we have strenuous jobs in the morning soon after sunlight, as our farmer ancestors did (and my family does), it's OK to eat breakfast. Otherwise, if we wake up hours after sunlight and have a sedentary morning, it is OK to just hydrate with water until we feel the *real* hunger, probably around late morning or noon. We should also eat smaller portions, preferably in smaller dishes like bowls, at a slower pace, pause and if still *really* hungry, make more than one trip to the kitchen. This allows us to work a little for the food we eat and minimize our brain's tendency to overindulge.

Stomach pains, acid refluxes (heartburns), smelly burps, constipation or loose stools (diarrhea), nausea, fatigue, brain fog or headaches, are all signs of improper food or eating habits. In the next chapter, In Chapter 2, I will share more body signs and biomarkers that can reveal the state of our inner metabolic balance.

There is no universal "best food" because we each have our unique metabolic needs, immune systems and constitutions. But we can have some rules of thumb, which I will share in this book. For starters, my oversimplified advice I shared in *The Rogue Brain* is:

"*Protein is for muscle work and signals our body for growth (of both muscles and cancer cells!) so it serves young people and anyone using a lot of muscles. Complex carbohydrates are for those who need more endurance than strength, like joggers or people who walk or climb a lot or for long hours. Small amounts of simple carbohydrates and fats are for those who do a lot of brain work (the best source would be chemical-free wild fruits and nuts). Vegetables, grains (like barley and oat), beans and starch (like chemical-free potatoes and rice) are for everyone.*"

Ancient cultures (China, Persia, India and Greece), however, considered each person's body as a mass and energy exchanger with its ecosystem. Physicians like Avicenna (10th century, from Persia, named *Ibn Sina* in local language) and Galen (2nd century, from Greece) who had no access to modern microscopes, MRIs or genetic sequencing, successfully treated diseases by *balancing the whole body* with food and medicine (purified natural substances). They stated that unlike objects without a soul (non-living), the human body, like all living systems, can only be in a state of dynamic equilibrium which is constantly prone to instabilities (malaise and disorders). The goal of a physician or a dietician was to return the body close to its dynamic *homeostasis* (energy balance), not to patch the symptoms for temporary relief of pain or symptoms.

To understand that approach, I have been studying parts of Avicenna's "The Canon of Medicine" (*Ghanoon fi Teb*) which built upon Galen's body of knowledge. Their approach, which parallels some Ayurvedic principles in India, includes defining and characterizing the overall *energetic* temperament (constitution) of each person. This is related to what we call *base metabolism* today. They gauged someone's "cold" or "warm" metabolic temperament by observing "whole body" indicators such as their skin firmness, color or pallor, stool or urination habits and shape, temperature and feel of their skin in places like their fingertips, etc. People's temperaments were also categorized by their propensity in fluid retention (such as high blood pressure), and extracellular fluid build up (such as edema and inflammation) as "dry-natured" or "damp-natured." For example, a constipated person may be judged to be of cold and dry constitution. Each person's constitution is to some degree controlled by the climate in which s/he was born or raised, or moved from and the environment they currently live in. So the best diet for someone from Alaska (with ancestors born there) who has moved to Arizona, may be different from the best (balancing) diet for someone from Arizona (ancestors born there) now living in Alaska! Our bodies, like all other living organisms on this planet, are dynamic energy exchange media that adapt to their environments. The more denatured our lifestyles and food become, the more we become metabolically disjointed from other living energy exchangers within our natural ecosystem.

The whole-body metabolic approach characterized each food with its energetic effect on our body's constitution and energy. Foods were categorized as "warm-natured" or "cold-natured," depending on their contribution to the person's base metabolic state. For example, in traditional Persian medicine garlic belonged to the "warm and dry" food category and would be best suited to balance people in "cold and damp" seasons or with that type of constitution. In modern medicine, a *cold* constitution may correspond to low metabolic rates (hypothyroidism or low thyroid activity, as symptomized by weight gain, low metabolism, hair loss or dry hair, dry skin, etc.) and *damp* may refer to conditions like edema or inflammation with extracellular fluid build up (and high blood pressure). So in today's language, garlic may be a good metabolic balancer (healthy food) for people with slower metabolism, low thyroid activity, high inflammation and blood pressure. However, it might not be advisable for the minority of people who already have high metabolism or low inflammation. I have a full article on my Substack about garlic which describes some of its history and science, as well as advantages of chemical-free garlic over cheap sprayed garlic.

Here is a general list of foods that can balance our metabolic temperament and imbalances, as well as seasonal or environmental metabolic needs:

Warm and Moist: Figs, grapes, apples, carrots, berries, sesame, red beans, honey, chickpeas, turkey meat, butter, cream, eggs.

Warm and Dry: Mango, garlic, eggplant, orange, mint, oregano, onions, fats, parsley, leeks, dates, tea, persimmons, cinnamon, basil, turmeric, saffron, ginger, walnuts, horseradish, black seed (cumin or caraway), pepper, venison (deer meat), camel meat and hump, coconut, sodium salt, french fries (fried salted potato).

Moderate: Rice, beet, blackberries, wheat, coffee, lettuce, banana, jujube, chicory, cow's milk, partridge meat, kheer (rice pudding with milk and honey), baked potato.

Cold and Moist: Spinach, plums, pomegranate, purslane, cheese, okra, cucumber, tomato, potato (raw), apricot, squash, pumpkin, pears, peaches, watermelons, goat milk, yogurt, fish meat, dried whey protein.

Cold and Dry: Millet, tamarind, barley, corn, vinegar, rhubarb, cilantro, lime, cherry, medlar, mung bean, beef

Traditional physicians recommended balancing cold foods with warm ones, like cheese with walnuts, fish or beef with dates or honey, rice with cumin or caraway.

Discussing the traditional Asian approach to metabolic balance and health, including the traditional Indian (Ayurveda), Persian and Chinese medicine (food choices) is beyond the scope of this book. There are good books written in English that cover the topic like *Healing with Whole Foods* by Paul Pitchford and *Basic Principles of Ayurveda* by D. P. Sharma and S. K. Shastri. These books offer a lot of information, including some complex metaphysical and philosophical underpinnings of ancient medicine and food advice. I think the easy-to-understand guidelines I include in this book are simple and good starting points for you to begin your journey to eating and living well.

Chapter 2: How does Food Signal Our Body?

As discussed, our body is an intelligent energy transfer factory that converts the biochemicals in food to whatever it feels it needs the most. The reason most diet fads and extreme diets do not work is because our body constantly converts molecules: Fats to sugars, sugars to fat, both fats and sugars to energy storage units called glycogen, amino acids to muscles and to proteins needed by the immune system and our blood (as envelope carriers of other molecules), short chain soluble fibers to short chain fatty acids, etc.

In deciding the best path to metabolize food, our body gets its cues from its own energy and nutrient needs, and from the content of the food it consumes. Sensing the food starts with our tongue. We usually reject bitter tastes or those that our body rejects. Our tongue sensors and receptors called taste buds are conditioned by our ancestral, childhood and adult diet. When we say many Americans have a "sweet tooth," it technically means their sugar sensors on their tongue have become too tolerant (addicted) to the sugar component of foods. My ancestral background has made me more tolerant of sour and acidic flavors like fermented foods and not as tolerant to sugary foods so most desserts taste too sweet to me and I avoid them.

The Standard American Diet (SAD) is often loaded with sugar, fat and salt. These flavors dull our senses over time because they may please our brain but not our body's metabolic needs. Like all other tolerances and addictions, our brain plays a role in our habits. We can sharpen our senses of taste and smell, and recondition our taste buds and preferences by changing our food habits and retraining our brain. This is discussed in detail in *The Rogue Brain.*

Once the brain receives taste and smell signals it triggers the increased production of saliva and gastric juices (from the stomach and pancreas). The relative ratios of macronutrients in the bloodstream like fats, proteins, sugars and fibers are also constantly evaluated by the brain to trigger the release of insulin or glucagon. Insulin is an *anabolic*, and glucagon a *catabolic* hormone. What does that mean?

Basically, hormones tell our body what to do with the *energy* and nutrients it collects from the food. The body has four major metabolic choices which I call the 4B's of Metabolism: Break down, Bury, Build or Burn. *Anabolic* hormones like insulin and testosterone (male reproductive and competitive/winning hormone) are anabolic so they signal the cells to absorb the excess energy sources in the blood to *Build* (muscles, fat cells, glycogen) or *Burn*. *Catabolic* hormones like glucagon and cortisol, released in times of stress, fasting, feeling cold, or after eating food higher in fat or protein than sugar or starch, signal the cells to *Break down* energy reserves (Fat, glycogen and muscles in extreme cases) to release more energy sources into the blood.

Insulin signaling in the brain regulates our appetite, as well as fat and amino acid metabolism in fatty (adipose) tissues and liver. If we keep eating when our body is not really starving for calories (*real* hunger), or consume too much simple sugars (which trigger insulin), our brain and body will ignore insulin signaling and become insulin-resistant. Our body will then accumulate fat even in places like the liver and muscles. Fat is our body's long-term storage of energy, for example when the brain expects a long winter and deficiency of caloric food (as in Alaska, and seen in bears) or in women of child-bearing age (through the action of estrogens) who may need to share that stored energy with a baby for a while. *Accumulated fat* is a necessity during long periods of caloric deficiency. In all other cases, excessive eating and calories (fat or sugars) in the diet is not what our body needs. Most natural, unprocessed food (not genetically-modified) without chemical additives and treatments would not trigger insulin resistance because they would not have excessive (unnatural, man-made) ratios of fibers, fat, carbs and protein.

If our diet is too lean on complex carbohydrates, like those in potatoes, oats and barley, and too rich in fats and proteins, or if we are stressed or starved for a while, the body releases *catabolic* hormones like cortisol and glucagon to break down our fat and glucose storage (like glycogens). This may be occasionally beneficial, for example when we have excess fat and our sedentary morning jobs do not use up much physical energy. In this case, we are better off going hungry to allow the catabolic hormones to use up some of our stored fat and glycogens before we eat more calories (and activate insulin). This is the concept behind time-restricted eating, for example between 11 AM and 6 PM, and involves skipping breakfast or late dinners. As with other one-size-fits-all diet fads, time-restricted eating is not for everyone. Obviously, if someone has a physically demanding job (calorie consuming) or a lean body, they may not benefit from time-restricted eating or ketogenic diets (see next).

Temporary physical stressors such as sauna or cold baths and certain diets called "ketogenic," that are rich in fats and low in carbohydrates can also trigger a catabolic (fat burning) mode in our body, called ketosis, which helps forms ketones in the blood as the main fuel for our cells (instead of glucose). *Autophagy*, which literally means "self-eating", can also be triggered by this diet, and allows the body to cannibalize waste products, toxic proteins and possibly cancerous cells. But here again, balance should be our goal. Excessive Break down (catabolic) mode, chronic or prolonged stress, starvation or carbohydrate (caloric) deficiency in diet and conditions like Type I diabetes (insufficient insulin), may lead to breaking down our valuable healthy muscles and tissues which are particularly valuable in aging populations, and in extreme cases to a condition called *ketoacidosis* which is dangerous.

I personally use a starchy low-sugar diet of fibrous vegetables or grains (potato, barley), some protein and fat but avoid extremely high-fat or high-protein diets. Once you train your mind and body to eat only when *really* (catabolically) hungry, you can even correlate your weight to your physiological appetite. I have noticed my fasting body weight, after waking up and urinating but before drinking or eating, closely tracks my real (catabolic) physiological hunger the night before. If I feel 95-99% full when I stop eating dinner (around 6 PM) I keep my steady weight the next morning regardless of how much or what I eat in my feeding window of 11:30 AM- 6:30 PM (except extra salty or sugary food which can lead to water retention and weight gain). Between hand cultivating our regenerative vegetable farmette, walking and occasional aerobic cardio (elliptical) machines, I burn additional calories a week, high enough to burn the desserts I like to enjoy, but low enough not to induce too much catabolic stress and hunger. Choosing proper activities, foods and eating habits and times, will help us balance our metabolic needs with the food we eat. There are no universal rules on how many calories and what type of calories we should consume. We just need to make sure we are neither fatigued nor burned out and have enough energy for a vital body, a sharp mind and a kind and patient soul.

Another component of metabolic efficiency, besides reducing psychological stressors in life, is to use food that adapts us to stresses by regulating the stress-induced inflammations or boosting our immune system. Chemical-free herbs and adaptogens such as turmeric, ginger, ginseng, garlic, onions, astragalus, ashwagandha, reishi, holy basil, fennel, arctic root (Rhodiola rosea) are potent regulators of our immune system. Herbs should be used cautiously and sparingly because they are naturally potent. For example, ashwagandha may increase the sedative effects of benzodiazepine drugs such as Valium, Ativan, Xanax, and other depressants. It has been shown that adaptogens have a mild prolonged stimulatory effect (vigilance, energy) on the body that reduces stress overloads and the ensuing exhaustion and fatigue because many adaptogenic herbs have chemical structures similar to the stress hormone adrenaline.

Apart from the form of energy available in the food, its composition also impacts our body's metabolism. The main types of building blocks in food, and what each does for our body, are outlined next.

Major Building Blocks in Foods

We have learned that each food sends a different metabolic signal to our brain, which prompts our metabolic factories to convert biochemicals to each other and to energy. Now we need to review the major building blocks (molecules) in foods that are responsible for metabolic changes in our body.

Amino Acids: These molecules help us build proteins, muscle and tissue cells (and their DNA which stores the blueprint), enzymes, neurotransmitters needed for proper functioning of our nervous system and brain, and other molecules needed by our immune system and our blood (as carriers of other molecules). Meats, beans and legumes are rich sources of amino acids but animal based amino acids like methionine in meat or leucine in dairy or meat, are particularly strong in promoting cellular proliferation pathways in our body, like one called the mTOR pathway, which promotes *growth of all cells, including cancer cells*! This is why meat and dairy may be more suitable for 7-30 year olds, including teenagers, children and young athletic adults in need of muscular, bone and cellular growth, than for middle-aged adults (30-60 years of age) that may be starting to host some cancer cells in their bodies. For children younger than 7 or adults older than 60, consumption of meat and dairy protein could have both benefits (in muscular growth) and downsides (in terms of suppression of their immune system). I will discuss good sources of meat, dairy and vegetables (to balance meat and dairy) later in the book.

There has been a lot of debate about our need for meat and dairy proteins vs. vegetable-based proteins. Generally speaking, middle-aged vegetarians who are not in muscularly-demanding lifestyles or jobs, can probably get their essential amino acid and protein needs from a vegetarian diet if they also consume some eggs and dairy (for lacto-ovo vegetarians), and certain grass-type or seed-type produce like quinoa, buckwheat, hemp seeds, chia seeds or spirulina.

Meat and dairy proteins are strong *anabolic* (Build) agents in our body and may be essential for certain people who suffer from wasting syndrome and cannot build muscle or fat tissues. Our muscles, for extra strength and endurance, rely on a molecule called Creatine which is easily converted to energy in times of exhaustion. Creatine is synthesized in our body from three amino acids which are abundant in meat (glycine, methionine, and arginine). Vegetarians tend to have lower amounts of creatine in their muscles.

Ancient Asian cultures assigned a different metabolic nature to each type of meat depending on its interaction with our metabolism because digestion and living are both energy transfer mechanisms. Beef for example, is fibrous and requires energy to break down and digest its proteins and fiber (even if marinated in acids like vinegar or lemon juice in advance) so it was assigned a "cold nature" in Asian medicine and should be balanced in the diet with "warm-natured" foods like dates, honey, walnuts or pepper, which are energy-positive and help our body not waste too much of its own energy in digesting the meat. Lamb, on the other hand, has a warmer nature because it has less muscle fibers, and more fat content that would supply our body with the calories needed to break down and digest the meat. Ancient Persian or Chinese medicine used the metabolic nature of the food to balance the metabolic constitution of the person (high or low energy).

Protein metabolism produces ammonia as a toxic by-product, which is converted by the liver to urea, and eliminated from the blood through the kidneys and excreted in urine. Uric acid, which is also a metabolite of meat, can trigger gout and aggregation of red blood cells, thickening of blood and an increased risk of heart attack. Methionine in meat metabolizes to sulfuric acid which like other meats and many medicines generally acidifies our blood and could lead to kidney stones and other metabolic disorders and diseases.

Carbohydrates: Carbs are great sources of energy in nature and our body. Complex carbohydrates like starches have long molecules and take longer to break down and release their energy in our body, if not boiled or baked. *Whole* grains and breads (if not from finely ground flour) have complex carbohydrates packed with fibers that *slowly* release the energy in our body, so they don't cause spikes in our blood sugar and a sudden rush of energy followed by fatigue. Most finely processed foods today lack the combination of fibers and complex carbohydrates so they can lead to insulin resistance. Simple sugars in food include fructose in fruits, glucose and polysaccharides in vegetables and lactose in milk. Upon sensing glucose in the blood, our brain orders release of insulin to signal our cells to start absorbing it from the blood. Glucose and insulin strongly influence growth of both normal and tumor cells because they activate the mTOR pathway already discussed.

Most fruits and vegetables today have been cross-hybridized or genetically modified to be sweeter (more fructose) and less fibrous. Fructose is the type of sugar which is difficult for our body to burn so without enough fiber that allows its slow release in our guts, it could disrupt our metabolism[5]. I like heritage heirloom chemical-free (non sprayed) apples that are smaller, more fibrous and sour, less sweet and not perfect-looking[6]! Commercially produced apples, like most other fruits, have been denatured and imbalanced in many ways and could cause metabolic imbalances in our body.

Fibers: These are long carbon chains found in cell walls and stems of vegetables and muscles of animals. Fibers are either soluble in water and our blood, like those in natural (not genetically modified) fruits, vegetables, whole grains and beans, or insoluble (roughage) and pass through our digestive tract to bulk up our stool. Insoluble fibers also bind sugar and fat molecules and allow them to release slowly in our guts. Soluble fibers are absorbed in our blood but also fermented by the beneficial bacteria in the lining of our gut to produce beneficial short-chain fatty acids that act like our gut's barrier against passage of toxins and undigested food particles into the bloodstream. Short chain fibers are sometimes called "prebiotic" because they are food to our "probiotic" (life-giving) gut bacteria. Our guts are called our "second brain" because they are innervated by the second largest neural network in our body (after our brain), including the all-important vagus nerve that controls our body's signal to our brain to allow relaxing (parasympathetic reaction following removal of stressful stimuli) and healing. Our guts also host the largest bacterial colony in our body, and are responsible for

---

[5] High fructose sweeteners are linked to metabolic syndromes/diseases.

[6] I have an article on Substack on "The Quest for Perfect-Looking Apple"

making serotonin, the body's important modulator of the immune system, metabolic balance, mood and motility in the digestive tract.

Unfortunately, most mass-produced food today of the processed, genetically-modified, chemically sprayed or fumigated type lack the beneficial combination of *good fiber and bacteria.* Again, denaturing our food for short-term economic benefits (Off-season availability, unnaturally long shelf lives and delivery distances, perfect looks and sweeter taste, low cost and high yield) is short-sighted because it disrupts the natural (raw) ratios of nutrients which our metabolism has adapted to over thousands of years. For example, sugars in nature are often pre packed with the minerals, enzymes, fibers and bacteria needed to metabolize it. We denature and imbalance our food, then spend a good part of our lives and resources to treat diseases caused by these imbalances.

Fats and Oils: Fats and oils are mostly acids with long hydrocarbon chains (tails) that make them dislike water (hydrophobic). When fatty acids and oils react with glycerol (glycerine) they form a dense fatty substance called triglyceride (TG). This is the type of fat in our blood that we don't want. Fats are also broken down in our body (or produced from glucose or body's energy reserves in times of glucose deficiency), and released into the blood together with protein carriers (remember, many proteins act as carriers in the blood) as High Density or Low Density Lipoproteins, called HDL or LDL cholesterols, respectively. HDL is called "good" cholesterol because it helps transport excess fat from the bloodstream to the liver, where it can be excreted from the body. LDL, however, brings cholesterol to the arteries, where it can accumulate and increase the risk of heart disease so LDL is called the "bad" cholesterol. Excessively high levels of LDL and TG in the blood are dangerous, but remember cholesterol is the building block for many of our hormones so depending on our hormonal needs, we may need more or less cholesterol. That is why athletes, teenegers and women may benefit more from cholesterol than others. Recent studies show that it is in fact the *ratio* of these fat types in the blood that matters the most for our metabolic health and balance. For example, a ratio of TG/HDL or LDL/HDL of less than 2 in blood test results is considered optimal.

As already discussed, ketogenic (high fat, low carbs) diets trigger a catabolic response in our body which could have benefits and risks. More important than the amount of fat in our diet, is the type of fat and how denatured it is. All fats and oils, such as seed oils, which are extracted, concentrated, heated or purified can be subject to oxidative damage and become harmful to our body. Certain oils like olive oil, *if cold-pressed fresh* (not heat or solvent-extracted) from chemical-free olives and kept in dark bottles and cold places, may resist oxidation and can be used sparingly in salads.

Butter from raw unpasteurized milk may contain some of the milk's beneficial lactobacilli bacteria (fermentation facilitator), Vitamins D and K2, which could help our body digest the butter fats. Nevertheless, even high quality raw butter should be used sparingly with food or for cooking (at medium but not high temperatures) because it's a purified and concentrated food (as we will see in Chapter 3).

Intramuscular fat (marble) is common in beef raised on corn or grains – as opposed to pasture-raised on grass. Certain nutritionists believe animal fat increases blood viscosity and sludge. Animal fats are generally not optimum fuels for our body to burn because of a metabolically damaging process called lipid peroxidation (inside our cells). When consumed in its natural state, however, the acetyl carnitine in meat can be helpful in metabolizing the fat inside our body and the fibers could slow down the release of fat cells into our cells and bloodstreams. Consuming fibers from vegetables is also helpful in not overwhelming our gastrointestinal (GI) with hard-to-metabolize fat cells.

Micronutrients: Unlike macronutrients mentioned so far, micronutrients are usually smaller molecules but because of their critical role in metabolizing the macronutrients without stressing our body, and their smaller quantities available in foods they are in some ways more precious and valuable than macronutrients. Micronutrients include minerals (such as calcium, potassium, magnesium, phosphorus, iodine, selenium and zinc), vitamins and antioxidants like polyphenols which are a plant's defense system against oxidative stress and damage and can help us with the same. The color of polyphenols and antioxidants seems to be an indicator of the portion of the electromagnetic energy spectrum they handle as part of the plant's metabolism and energy dissipation.

Vitamins are either fat-soluble like vitamins A, D, E, and K, which are abundant in dairy and eggs and can be stored in our body and accumulate over time if not needed, or water-soluble like vitamins B and C, the excess of which are excreted into the blood and then urine so they are not stored in the body and must be consumed regularly. Each vitamin has a specific function in the body.

Vitamin A, which is in carrots and the orange colored pigments you see in grass-fed milk and free-ranging chicken eggs, is important for vision, immune function, and skin health.

Vitamin C is essential for immune function, wound healing, and collagen production, and mainly found in vegetables, plants and fruits. As a result, the same way a meat-based diet could offer a person stronger muscles and faster growth, a vegan diet could offer a person more endurance, recovery, healing and protection against diseases like cancer.

Vitamin D mainly helps with calcium metabolism so it is crucial for bone health and immune function. Our own body can make it from Cholesterol type molecules (from fat) with proper exposure to sunlight. It's also available in unpasteurized raw dairy and in concentrated form in cod liver oil. Vitamin D is involved in so many vital functions of the human body that Henry Lahore, founder of VitaminDWiki has dedicated a whole website to these functions. I cannot endorse or verify claims on supplements but I find the science about vitamin D interesting and educational.

Vitamin E acts as an antioxidant to protect cells from damage. It's available in animal and vegetable-based foods as well as nuts and seeds..

Vitamin K is necessary for proper blood clotting (not too much and not too little). Vitamin K1 found in vegetables, seems to be a lot less potent in calcium metabolism and bone health than vitamin K2, which is found in animal products (raw milk and egg yolks) and fermented food like kefir, natto and sauerkraut. Vitamin K2 helps the calcium which is delivered by Vitamin D into our bloodstream deposit in the right places in the body like in bones and teeth, and not in wrong places like the kidney, eyes (cataract), or arteries. Vitamin K2 can also disrupt cancer cell growth cycles. High heat Pasteurization of raw milk destroys bacteria producing Vitamin K2.

B vitamins play a role in energy production, nerve function, heart, skin and tissue health. The only B vitamin which is not abundant in commercial (unfermented) vegetables is Vitamin B12, required as a cofactor in DNA synthesis, and for the synthesis of myelin sheaths covering our nerves, and in maturation of red blood cells in the bone marrow. Vitamin B12, also known as cobalamin, is structurally similar to hemoglobin in red blood cells and chlorophyll in green plants, except it has cobalt as its central atom (vs. iron in hemoglobin and magnesium in chlorophyll). B12 is exclusively produced by certain soil microbes that live in symbiotic relationships with plant roots, and gut bacteria in humans and animals (cows rumens). Vegetarians who do not include dairy, fish and eggs in their diet, are at a high risk of vitamin B12 deficiency, especially if they consume unfermented vegetables from sprayed soil. Similar to animal-based proteins, vitamin B12 deficiencies have a greater effect on children, pregnant women and elderly people who are more reliant on cellular growth pathways.

Polyphenols and antioxidants are compounds available in fruits and vegetables to protect them against stressors (thermal or hydration) and injuries (by bugs and animals). They are believed to impart some of these benefits to the humans eating them too (in moderation). Like vitamin C, polyphenols are more abundant in vegetarian diets.

Calcium: It is an all-important mineral that plays many roles in our body. Our bones are the largest reserves of calcium which is metabolized by its cofactors: magnesium, potassium, sodium and Vitamins K2 (see above) and D in performing functions such as neuronal signaling, blood coagulation, platelet adhesion and contraction of myocardial (heart), smooth muscles and blood vessels – called vasoconstriction in times of stress or infectious injury. Too much calcium in the diet not balanced by its cofactors, or released by the body's stress response (by breaking down our bones and teeth) may lead to neurological, heart, muscular or eye diseases, kidney stones or constipation.

Magnesium: It is a mineral which seems to be nature's balance to calcium. If too much calcium constipates us or makes our muscles and blood vessels tight and our heart beating faster, too much magnesium can induce diarrhea, relaxation, and low blood pressures. Magnesium deficiency is common in metabolic disorders such as obesity, type 2 diabetes, and insulin resistance. These disorders are also associated with a high incidence of cancer. Researcher Harry Rubin calls magnesium the "regulator par excellence of metabolism," largely through its role as a cofactor for ATP and phosphoryl transfers inside our cells as explained in Chapter 5. Magnesium is mostly found in the Chlorophyll in green leaves of plants and vegetables In fact, there is a striking resemblance between structures of hemoglobin in red blood cells delivering oxygen to living cells, and Chlorophyll in green leaves, generating and delivering oxygen to plants. In their core, hemoglobin has iron and chlorophyll has magnesium for energy and electron transfer. In fact, anemic people seem to benefit from wheatgrass and other chlorophyll-rich diets. I find this as another little-studied secret of creation and evidence of the continuity and symbiosis of the energy transfer chain on this planet between animals and vegetables.

Sodium and Potassium: Sodium in table salt is another purified and concentrated food denatured from its natural state, which is often with water and balanced with other minerals like potassium and magnesium. Unrefined salts such as those from Celtic or Himalayan caves may offer a better balance of potassium to sodium. This balance is important because our body relies on the sodium and potassium exchanges across our cell (plasma) membranes including cardiac (heart) tissue, neurons, and in the kidney. Too much purified sodium (as in table salt) not balanced by potassium leads to high blood pressures, headaches, thirst, swollen feet and hands, dark urine and irregular heartbeats. Generally speaking, if the body's electrolytes (sodium, potassium, calcium and magnesium) are imbalanced, it may disrupt cellular functions across the body from nervous system, to digestive tract and our heart (irregular heartbeats). This is yet another reason to use food which is as close as possible to its biochemically balanced form in nature. Purified salts and minerals, and heavily-fertilized, non-organic vegetables grown in pesticides-sprayed fields are denatured.

Iron: It is needed in small amounts by our body because most of it is recycled (not wasted) after old red blood cells are excreted. Women who menstruate or people who lose blood can benefit from iron (ideally not from supplements to avoid toxic overload). Iron is a vital nutrient for virtually all forms of life because of its role in cellular processes ranging from energy generation and DNA replication to oxygen transport (in red blood cells). But bacterial pathogens also use their host's iron in order to replicate and cause disease so excessive iron can make us prone to infectious diseases. Heme iron, the type of iron found predominantly in animal products like meat, is more bioavailable than other types of iron. Females and people on raw vegetarian diets may be more prone to anemia than meat eaters. But as stated, having too much iron could be dangerous in pathogenic environments. In fact, anemia and conditions like sickle cell disease may be considered as the human body's intelligent adaptive strategy to protect us in infectious environments from dangerous bacteria (as in malaria) by depriving them of the iron they need to grow.

Human-friendly Bacteria like lactobacillus are often not listed among micronutrients but I include them here because they are probably the single most important missing element in our modern diets. Vegetables, fruits and nuts which are sprayed for insects and weeds, fumigated for shelf life and appearance and sometimes wax-coated, irradiated or gassed, look perfect and unspoilable because they are not appealing to any living organisms, which unlike humans, know the right way to eat. Unlike other living organisms, humans are not preprogrammed to instinctually select good food which balances us. Fermented foods made with raw, chemical-free and good quality ingredients should be part of our regular diet to improve our gut health, immune system and metabolic balance. See the explanation already provided under "Fibers" about the crucial role of good bacteria in regulating our nervous and immune system.

Our Body's Telltale Signs About Food

This is not a book about physiology so if you are seeking medical advice, you should consult with an integrative or functional medicine practitioner. To understand the compatibility of any food to our metabolic needs, however, we need to assess its impact on our overall health. There are some inexpensive "whole body" feedback signals which are telltale signs of the beneficial or harmful nature of our food. As discussed in the previous section, before the age of expensive organ-level diagnostic tools, ancient physicians relied on whole body signals to decide how to metabolically balance a person using food or medicine (often purified natural herbs, similar to today's natural vitamins, herbal supplements or tinctures).

In the human body, there are many signals that correlate well with the body's overall level of balance and health – technically called *homeostasis* as I explained in my previous books. We have to relearn how to listen to these signs to see what our food is doing to our body:

Motion (kinesthetics): Restricted motions caused by body pains such as arthritis, may be related to mineral metabolism (calcium, potassium, sodium, magnesium), the body's stress response (sympathetic), or chronic inflammation caused by denatured/processed food. We have discussed balancing calcium metabolism and reducing inflammations elsewhere in the book.

Behaviors: Being short-tempered or uptight may be associated with high blood pressure, constipation, gut issues, sleep disorders and sexual dysfunctions, all possibly resulting from the body's stress response (sympathetic) and mineral metabolism (calcium, potassium, sodium, magnesium balance). In my last two books, I discussed the cerebral (brain) roots of the issue. In this book, I will discuss the dietary roots of the problem.

Urine: The frequency, volume, color, turbidity and pH of your urine all reveal the state of your metabolic balance. For example, the balance of sodium and potassium in your diet and body, the amount of water in your diet, your body's stress response, and blood pressure control the volume of the urine. Darkish yellow colors and thick consistency (viscosity) may indicate dehydration or protein in the urine. Acidic pH below 6.5 may indicate oxidative stress and a poor diet low in vegetables that can trigger kidney stones. You can use an inexpensive pH meter on an occasional basis to assess your urine's pH.

Stool Habits and Excrement: Again, the frequency, morphology (shape and structure), color, dryness and density are all telltale signs of your food metabolism. Constipation and disorders in stool habits, also usually associated with body's stress response (sympathetic) and mineral metabolism (calcium, potassium, sodium, magnesium balance), are early but important signals for several diseases, including kidney stones, heart disease, cataract and sexual dysfunctions.

Sweat: Sweating is our body's natural mechanism to cool us down, and remove toxins and excess electrolytes from the body. Excess sweating may relate to hormonal imbalances (like thyroid and cortisol), and the pungent ammonia-like smell may relate to bad bacteria or the amount of meat and protein (high-nitrogen foods) we consume. Good bacteria like those in fermented food, and low-protein diets can help reduce the odor. Some deodorants now contain good (lactobacillus) bacteria to fight sweat odors in people lacking these bacteria in their body and diet.

Skin: Too many brown and acne spots, and slow healing indicate imbalances in diet and hormones (like thyroid), and disorders in sleep and digestion. Skin elasticity and turgor (internal cellular pressure that prevents a wilted wrinkled look) especially under chins and eyes and on our neck and dorsal (back) side of our hands indicate vitality, which decreases with age, dehydration and bad diet. Pallor and yellowness relate to the low ratio of red blood cells and bilirubin in the blood, which relate to our liver dysfunctions, poor sunlight exposure and diets high in fat and protein.

Cravings: If they are not cravings of the brain (for sugar, salt and fat), they can tell us about our body's deficiencies. For example, it is now evident that a strong craving for chewing ice (called pagophagia) is associated with iron deficiency. Our other cravings can also be linked to our mineral or hormonal imbalances. For example, "Geophagia" which refers to craving and eating dirt, common during pregnancy and childhood, could indicate deficiency in minerals like zinc or the need to bind harmful toxins in our GI tract by clay-like dirt. Pica is a generic term that refers to craving for non-food items. Although the medical industry treats it as a disorder, it is rooted in our body's deficiency of important nutrients missing in the low quality, commercially produced food we consume. It's our body talking to us, and begging us for what it really needs.

Hair and Nails: Brittleness and slow growth again indicate imbalances in diet and hormones (like thyroid), disorders in sleep and stool/digestion and poor exposure to sunlight.

Vitality, Energy and Patience: A balanced diet gives us the energy and passion to play in nature, as opposed to a constant inclination to stay indoors and sedentary, to learn and be curious, and to have fellowship and friendship (non work-related) with other humans without resorting to crutches like energy drinks, coffee, alcohol, electronics, drugs, smokes, etc. In other words, a good diet brings out our inner child, the time of our life when we were metabolically more balanced.

Libido and Reproductive Health: Intimate loving relations and sexual satisfaction/functions when married can be indicators of a balanced diet, metabolism and blood flow. The physiology of blood flow to reproductive organs is mediated by nitric oxide, the messenger molecule for vasodilation (expanding of blood vessels), which is also linked to cellular growth, insulin metabolism, relaxation, immune response and cardiovascular health. We already discussed how the good bacteria in our mouth and on the leaves of lettuce help us chew and release nitric oxide. Chronic stress response can not only constipate us but also increase our blood pressure and impact our reproductive health because it depletes acetylcholine, the neurotransmitter manufactured in our body from food, that signals vascular cells to produce nitric oxide.

Weight and Appetite Changes: There should be little if any changes in our weight and appetite from day to day if we have a good and balanced diet and lifestyle factors such as regular sleep/eating times, exposure to sunlight and physical activity, and if we minimize our psychological stresses imposed by our unruly brain.

****

Besides these whole-body signals and biomarkers, diseases can tell us a lot about the destiny of our food inside our body. For example, kidney stones, mostly of the calcium oxalate type, indicate improper metabolism of oxalates and calcium in the body. Calcium belongs to bones, our nerves (for signaling) and in our neuromuscular junctions, and not in the arteries or kidney. Oxalates are found in large quantities in spinach, dark leafy greens, tea, nuts, chocolate, or formed when proteins, ascorbic or amino acids are metabolized. It now appears that some or all of the following factors can lead to the dysfunction in the metabolism of calcium and oxalate: Sedentary lifestyles, lack of mobility, high sodium and protein diets, high blood pressure, acidic urine (already discussed), stress, low exposure to sunlight, pasteurized milk and dairy devoid of the natural Vitamin K and D needed for calcium metabolism (On Simplescience.Substack.com you can find my article on this topic), unhealthy gut bacteria from processed and unfermented food made from sprayed or denatured ingredients, low water intake, low consumption of citrus fruits, as well as diets too rich in protein, salt, chocolate, spinach and other oxalate-containing food, plus some genetic disposition or history of kidney stones, etc.

Interestingly, many of these factors have also been implicated in coronary heart disease, cataract, arthritis and other metabolic disorders involving the calcium metabolism loops in the body. Our metabolic health is indeed an *interconnected* "whole-body" function, which involves *all* organs and all the food ingredients broken down in our body (metabolites). So different diseases are basically different manifestations (symptoms) of a dysfunctional metabolism in our body. Unhealthy organs are like the weakest links that break first in a collapsing unstable network. Eating and living well supports our healthy metabolic network. But when the links in that network start to break, the current science and business of medicine with its *reductionist* approach[7] can only try to

---

[7] I explain *reductionism* in my first book *Masks, Crutches and Daggers*

patch up the broken links (organ, disease, protein, etc.) separately and one at a time.

Generally speaking, good food delivers essential building blocks to our body without disrupting its natural flows. For example, foods, medicines or hormones that thicken or thin our blood too much, and increase or decrease its viscosity excessively could lead to heart diseases or strokes. Too much fat, sugar, salt and animal protein can impact our blood viscosity and its healthy flow to the heart and brain.

Too much fiber can disrupt our gut functions and the normal flow of food in our digestive tract. Certain weight control medicines try to simulate this effect. Too much fiber also increases the viscosity and bulk volume of our stool (digested food residue not absorbed by the blood in the small intestine) while too little fiber reduces the poop's bulk volume. Using a "toothpaste" analogy, for proper flow and squeezing it out from the tube you don't want the paste to be too dry but you don't want it to be too sticky or runny!

The amount and type of fiber in the food, along with its water, fat and mineral content, control its flow in our colons. Drugs that disrupt our metabolic pathways (by regulating our blood sugar, insulin or weight) can disrupt our digestive health. For example, popular drugs like Metformin and Ozempic are known to cause serious gastrointestinal disorders, diarrhea or nausea in many patients by interfering with their digestion rate and carbohydrate metabolism. The natural process of digestion relies on releasing the energy in food (like the starch in chemical-free potatoes) to our body. The more we denature that process and upset the natural balances (and ratios) of ingredients from what is in their natural form, the more likely it is for the food to be disruptive to our metabolism. In fact, in the next Chapter, we discuss the important concept of *denaturation* and *adulteration.*

Chapter 3: Denaturation and Adulteration Score

As we learned so far, food in its natural form, not denatured or adulterated by humans, if consumed in moderation and when our body really craves for it, will cause little or no stress on our body's metabolic health (homeostasis and equilibrium). Protein, for example, in natural meat form, is diluted and balanced by fibers in the connecting collagen and gristle tissues, and by fat which is metabolized in our body by acetyl carnitine in the meat. In addition, meat, pasture-raised on natural grasslands will have the orange-colored beta carotene (precursor to vitamin A) in its fat layers which would help with cleaner metabolism of meat and fat. Fruits and vegetables are no different. Oranges and apples are packaged by nature with a lot of fiber, such as pectin, which balances fructose and slows down its release into our blood to prevent blood sugar spikes. In contrast, pure human-made concentrated forms of food like protein powders or fruit juices (without fibers) will not be as naturally and efficiently metabolized by our body. Most denatured food is low quality food. In my view, the *quality* of food we eat, in terms of its *metabolic contribution* to our body, is more important than the quantity, appearance, cost or type of food we eat.

Every time we disrupt the natural state of any food by processing, denaturing and disjointing its compounds, we create deficiencies and imbalances in them and lower their metabolic quality. For example, salt in its most natural form is in a thermodynamically stable state in equilibrium with the water that contains it, as in sea water (around 97% water). Furthermore, sodium, potassium, calcium and magnesium balance each other in nature depending on their abundance and the environment, like the soil in which the vegetable grows in. When humans spend energy to disturb the minerals' natural equilibrium state, for example by evaporating sea water and removing minerals other than the purified and concentrated sodium salt (sodium chloride), a *thermodynamically-unstable* compound is created which will keep seeking water. Ancient sages and mystics did not know thermodynamics but were aware that force-separating anything from its natural and stable/balanced state would lead to metastable (or quasi-equilibrium) energy states. Jalāl al-Dīn Balkhi (Rumi), the esteemed 13th century Persian mystic opens his well-known *Mathnavi* with a beautiful poem about lamentations of anyone or anything in the universe torn asunder (separated) from its natural state, and yearning to join back the roots[8].

So purified sodium salt is very thirsty for water and will form a clump or cake with the slightest exposure to humidity. That is why commercial granulated salts often have anti-caking additives to prevent this. But forming clumps inside the package or inside the salt shakes in our kitchens is not the worst part of denaturing salt. The problems arise *inside* our body. When we consume purified (read imbalanced) sodium, it means it will seek a lot of water while inside our blood stream to get back to its natural state of (thermodynamic) balance. This is the so-called "antidiuretic" effect of salt in our body leading to high blood pressure caused by retaining too much water inside our bloodstreams and reducing our normal urine volume and flow. As mentioned earlier, unrefined and naturally-balanced salts (like pink cave salts with high potassium and less sodium) seem to be less disruptive to our water balance cycles and blood pressure because the minerals in these salts are closer to their natural and stable states.

Refined sea salt and many forms of solid food such as powdered egg, milk, spices, flour, sugar and many

---

[8] Although he uses a mystic language to refer to our soul's alienation from pure love and unison with others and the creator, he says disturbances always follow separation from a natural state..

modern pantry items are pulverized and milled to unnaturally *superfine* particle sizes, with a high surface area. Solids denatured this way tend to flocculate (scientific term for "lumping together") over time and resist free flowing. So my fellow engineers and scientists spend a lot of money and time to find ways to *unnaturally force unnaturally pulverized* powders to stabilize and not lump. One trick used is adding cheap anti-caking additives such as sodium aluminosilicate (as in powdered salt), sodium dioxide (as in powdered egg solids and beer filtrates), calcium silicate (as in powdered spices) or cellulose (as in grated parmesan cheese, and as wood pulp in diapers). In 2016 Walmart was sued for selling cans of 100% grated parmesan cheese that actually contained up to 10% cellulose (wood pulp) as an anti-caking additive. And the problem is not just the level of cheap anti-caking additives, but their impact on our health. Although many anti-caking additives are labeled by the FDA as GRAS (Generally Recognized As Safe) many can be harmful in high doses or if denatured. For example, the Aluminum in anti-caking additives is associated with Alzheimer's and other neurodegenerative diseases.

And it's not only salts, flours and sugars that are denatured. Most commercial mass-produced foods, even plants and animals, are extensively processed and adulterated to (A) Lower their cost, (B) Increase their shelf life, (C) Make them available outside the harvest or production season and in places far from the place of production, (D) Make them look good or perfect, (E) Increase their sugar or salt content, (F) Reduce their fiber and bran content, (F) Produce them in large scale with uniform packaging with low risk of contamination and spoilage. But every one of these goals, which is good for business and convenience[9] is usually bad for the food and our metabolism.

---

[9] What I call convenience, speed and scale in *The Rogue Brain*

In this chapter, I have come up with a subjective way to evaluate how far your food is removed from its natural, thermodynamically-stable "ground" state. Basically, we start from any food in its most natural, undisturbed state, the way it was before humans had a chance to make any changes. For example, for fish, it would be in clean rivers and oceans and not in fish farms made by humans. That ground state would have a score of 0 in our adulteration and denaturation chart. So for each of the following changes and processes, we *subtract* some points. The more negative the score, the farther removed it is from its natural balance and state:

Dehydration, water removal and partial drying up: -1

Complete dehydration: -2

Seasoning with salt, sugar or dehydrated spices: -1

Adding natural additives and preservatives: -2

Adding synthetics like flavors (like MSG) and colors: -3

Adding more than 5 ingredients: -1 for each additional

Genetic modification or engineering: -3

Grinding for granulation: - 1

Fine grinding and making powders: -2

Removing husks, brans or fibers: -2

Spraying in the field with pesticides: -3

Post-treatment like with waxes and fumigants: -3

Purification/extraction with water/natural solvents: -1

Purification/extraction with synthetic solvents: -2

Extraction with synthetic solvents plus HEAT: -3

Each additional stage of heating above 140 ℉: -2

Solids packaged in air-tight containers: -1

Liquids packaged in airtight plastics or plastic-coated paper or metal: -2

Transportation beyond 300 miles: -1 for each 200 miles

Shelf life beyond 3 months: -1 for each 6 months

Obviously, you need to educate yourself about the processing of your food before figuring out how negative its score is. For example, let's find the score for decaffeinated coffee. The coffee beans start as ripe cherries which are sprayed or fumigated (-6), followed by removal of the skin and the pulp (-2 for fiber removal), pulping and fermenting the beans, drying them (-1), milling and hulling (more fiber removed), roasting the beans at 400 ℉ (-2), Grinding them (-1, but -2 for fine grind like espresso), removing the caffeine (if using synthetic solvents like ethyl acetate or methylene chloride with heat, - 3, if using water extraction: -1), Brewing and extraction with water and heat (-2). So a typical decaffeinated cup of non-organic coffee has a denaturation score of -16 or even higher if from genetically-modified beans.

While we cannot be food purists, we can strive to grow some of our vegetables and herbs using chemical-free, hand-cultivated methods or buy them from smaller local farms that use these regenerative methods even if we have to travel to the countryside and look around. If you can find organic (chemical-free) whole grains, try to buy them in bulk, grind them fresh and in small quantities, and make your own whole-grain food. Some grains need to be dehulled for natural digestion by humans so dehulling is not part of denaturation for humans.

Avoid foods with denaturation scores of -8 or higher (in negativity). For example, typical orange juice in the store probably has an adulteration score of -15: Sprayed non-organic oranges (-3), juiced and removed fiber and pulp (-2), added sugar (-2), heated and packaged juice (-4), Transported from 1000 miles + (-4). But organic (non sprayed) fruits (not juiced) from a nearby state within 500 miles and in season would be a -1, a much better choice. And if you buy it from a local farmer less than 300 miles away, even better (perfect score)! Just 90 years ago, most people either made their own food (farming and raising animals) or bought it from sources within 100 miles, fresh, in season and not sprayed. Chemical pesticides became widespread after World War II when companies manufacturing chemicals for war turned some of that surplus capacity into making pesticides to stage a war against nature! In fact, chemicals like Agent Orange, used in Vietnam as an herbicide and defoliant, are seriously harmful to humans too. As discussed earlier, the chlorophyll of green plants and the hemoglobin of red blood cells in humans are biochemically similar.

One of the most denatured foods is sugar, which can be called the "sweet cocaine" due to its addictive effect on the human brain. It is dehydrated, heated, defibered, concentrated, bleached, milled to a powder so it is very far from its natural metabolic state balanced with water, fiber, probiotic bacteria and large particles. Other intensely sweet highly denatured forms of calories like the high fructose corn syrup can be addictive and also seriously harm our body's metabolic factories like our liver. Today, even fruits are cross hybridized or genetically modified to be artificially and unnaturally sweet and lacking the natural levels of fibers and seeds. Certain fruits like seedless grapes and melons are now contraindicated by doctors for diabetic or prediabetic patients due to these fruits' sugar content and triggering insulin resistance.

Another widely used and abused denatured concentrated drink is alcohol, which regardless of its form has a high adulteration score. Natural forms of alcohol found in fermented fruits for example, are below 1%, as compared to typical synthetic (denatured) alcoholic beverages that contain 10-20% alcohol. Metabolically speaking, our body really doesn't know what to do with concentrated alcohol, so that is why alcohol, as a fuel, initially causes vasodilation (relaxation of blood vessels), elevated metabolism, energy and sense of elation, followed at higher levels and time exposures by vasoconstriction (shrinking of blood vessels), headaches, low energy and hangover. The short term inhibitory effects of alcohol such as elation and reduction of anxiety, are followed by withdrawal – after consumption is reduced – to stress (nervousness, agitation) and therefore, dependence and addiction. Alcohol is not available in nature at high concentrations, and is a toxin to stem and progenitor cells, i.e., life. Its effect on our nervous system parallels that of Benzodiazepines' (an addictive anxiolytic drug)[10].

Generally speaking, a metabolically efficient diet is one closer to its natural form with minimal purification or processing. There are only a few natural processes which make food more metabolically efficient, such as slow fermentation. Fermented foods such as yogurt, sauerkraut, kimchi and kefir are a group of naturally processed foods that seem to be microbiologically beneficial for our metabolism and immune system, and make us less prone to metabolic and infectious diseases. As referenced in my website and social media blogs, we do quite a bit of fermentation with lactic-acid bacteria in our household using locally sourced, raw organic ingredients. Store brand fermented products limit the degree of fermentation because the ongoing anaerobic process could release too much carbon dioxide, which acidifies and destroys harmful pathogens but can also cause dangerous pressure build up in pre-packaged store brands. This is perhaps why store-brand Kombucha bottles are often made out of thick glass. Our

---

[10] Both alcohol and Benzodiazepines amplify the effect of neurotransmitter GABA so they initially reduce our neural activity and have a sedative effect but over time, once GABA receptors adapt and are desensitized, people feel agitated and less calm upon withdrawal.

home-made fermented foods are often sour, indicating the formation of a good amount of lactic or acetic acid which feed the beneficial probiotic microorganisms but prevent against most other microbes. Fermented foods such as kefir are now labeled as *psychobiotic* because they are shown in animal studies to signal through the microbiota-gut- immune-brain axis and positively modulate host behavior and immune system. Remember, a healthy gut, which scientists now call our "second brain" is essential for a healthy brain and good decisions, what our ancestors called "gut feelings."

The Least Denatured Forms of Food

Most processed and denatured food today have too little water, soluble fiber, probiotic bacteria and enzymes, magnesium and potassium. Instead they have high concentrations of ingredients like sugar, sodium salt, preservatives and color additives that help the food last longer in warehouses, trucks and stores, and look perfect on store shelves. We usually know a food is denatured when bugs and bees stay away from it. Here is a list of the least denatured forms of food:

Animal Proteins: A good source of protein is wild ocean-caught fish frozen and without too many preservatives and additives and no older than six months from date of catch, or catching your own fish if you are lucky or wise enough to have the time and can find uncontaminated waters – a rarity! – away from industrial or residential polluters. Other good protein sources are pasture-raised lamb or beef from naturally-born cows (*not AI, or artificially inseminated*), that grazed freely on chemical-free grasslands and prairies (not sprayed with pesticides), humanely treated and not stressed before or during the slaughter process. Most chicken meat and eggs are unfortunately produced in commercial settings that are extremely stressful to the animals (see below) so many people now avoid eating chicken meat, and only use *pasture-raised* eggs from organic or chemical-free farms.

Eggs: Eggs are an amazing source of vitamins and proteins. Most commercial egg factories expose chickens to extremely stressful conditions which cannot be healthy for them, for their eggs or for us. If you can raise your own free-ranging chickens humanely, it's wise to do so. The eggs will have an amazing taste and your chickens would be happy to be free ranging in a pasture or grassland while protected by you from predators. The orangish color of the egg yolk is an indication of the carotenoids (precursors to vitamin A) derived from the grass chickens feed on. The orange color of the cream in raw milk is also derived from cow's metabolizing grass into carotenoids. I include more details about eggs in a special section below.

Milk: Raw milk from grass-fed pasture-raised cows would have plenty of fat-soluble vitamins A, D, E and K plus calcium and protein. Some dairy farms expose cows to extremely stressful conditions which cannot be good for the cow, its milk and our health. There are also problems with pasteurization and homogenization which I explain in detail later in this chapter.

Oils and Fats: We do need some fat because vitamins like A, D, E and K are fat soluble. Yet, most oil and fatty acids, even those minimally processed/denatured, including seed oils and nut oils, gradually denature over time because of the effect of temperature, oxygen and light on their chemical structure (double bonds). Solid animal fats and butter may resist oxidation a bit longer but are still less than ideal sources of calories for regular human use because they are denatured.

Animal fats are separated from muscle tissue fibers and butter is separated from water and whey. Small amounts of "fresh" natural fats and oils, raw butter, and fat that is naturally attached to the meat protein listed above, which have not been overly processed, denatured or aged (oxidized) can be helpful in most people's diets especially women and youth with hormonal needs. Fats give us *satiety* and prevent us from overeating other food types. Fats are sometimes better metabolized when paired with meat, fruits or acidic food like vinegar or lemon juice. Many athletes use nuts and fruits as their healthy midday source of protein and fat between lunch and dinner. Sages like Mohandas Gandhi, leader of Indian dependence, relied mostly on fruits and nuts for their diet.

For salad dressing and to provide some lubrication for the roughage (insoluble fibers), we can use cold-pressed olive oil from organic (chemical-free) olives packaged in dark glass containers and stored cool or cold for no longer than six months. Generally speaking, deep fried salty food may be tasty but it is not a healthy source of energy, especially if smoke is rising from the superheated oil, or if the oil has been used multiple times or getting dark or viscous.

Vegetables, Herbs, Grains: These are great sources of vitamins A, B and C needed for healing, recovery and cellular protection against oxidative stress. Whenever possible buy vegetables, herbs and grains fresh from local small family farms that use regenerative chemical-free methods. Try buying whole grains like unbleached whole grain organic wheat in bulk and then grind smaller quantities at home for making your own bread on-demand at home. Sourdough bread takes longer to prepare but it makes the proteins and gluten in wheat more digestible for our body. The bran (outer layer) in whole grain wheat includes valuable nutrition and oils. Certain vegetables, if grown naturally and without chemicals, are among the most nutritious or healing foods out there. For example, potatoes are among the cheapest and best sources of starch and energy for humans. Potato's impressive high fiber content and nutrient density (Vitamins A, B and C, micronutrients, magnesium, phosphate, potassium, iron, copper, and calcium) make it a superfood for our cardiovascular and digestive health as well as immune system. Garlic, on the other hand, offers amazing therapeutic and healing properties. Herbs are potent and concentrated sources of micronutrients so they should be used sparingly to balance other foods and to heal us in times of imbalance.

For example, thyme has strong mucoactive properties, which means it stimulates mucosal activity in our respiratory tract and helps us clear it, which is beneficial to fight bacterial infections. This is how it works: Our nasal and respiratory passages and our mouth, release mucus that contains beneficial (friendly) bacteria and proteins called IgA (Immunoglobulin type A), a type of antibody in our immune systems and specialize in breaking down and destroying harmful bacteria, trapping them in the sticky and viscous mucus and preventing them from progressing deeper into our lungs. Good food ensures we have a strong and balanced immune system (such as the mucosal nasal and salivary IgA and good bacteria in our nose and mouth) which act as gatekeepers in our body's entrances of nose and mouth. Chemicals in food and medicine, alcohol and many mouthwashes, toothpastes and nasal sprays, and water with excessive fluoride or chlorine can harm our mucosal defense efficiency while herbs like thyme can enhance our mucosal defense. Historically, herbs have been used for their medicinal properties for a variety of diseases and disorders, internally or externally (our skin and hair). Some of today's expensive pharmaceutical compounds are in fact synthetic versions or derivatives of biochemically active molecules in herbs.

Fruits: Again, chemical-free, smaller and local orchards, and heirloom varieties which have not been sweetened, defibered or de-seeded (seedless) are better choices. Tasteless fruits that are waxed, fumigated, or picked unripe and then gassed to look ripe are not good choices. See the section of fruits and apples below.

The Foolish Quest for Perfect Fruits

The following few sections are modified excerpts of my full educational articles on my substack and website about food. This section is about how buying perfect-looking fruits in stores may not be the wisest thing to do. Such supermarket fruits look perfect but may have poor flavor and aroma, low fiber and probiotic bacteria levels, and high sugar content. I attribute the problem to the insane quest by modern humans to "quantify" quality:

As you may know by now (especially if you read my books and articles), the new species of humans I call *Homo economicus*, is a "*quantitatively*-driven" species which tirelessly pursues and monetizes "perfection" through expansion of scale (quantity), speed and convenience. And even his perception of "quality" is formed by physically "quantifying" it! For example, when it comes to apples, commercial producers classify the *quality* of apples by its *size* such as "Minimum 2.5 inch in diameter" or *degree of redness*. None of these *quantities* are necessarily indicators of quality if the fruit is harvested prematurely and gassed for color development, or if the variety has a naturally dull color.

So commercial "large-scale" apple growers go to great lengths such as using chemical pesticides, post-harvest gas chambers, and other non-regenerative mechanized approaches, to grow, harvest, sort, and package standard *size* apples of uniform color. This level of perfection and standardization is unnatural because nature follows spectral and biodiverse growth patterns, producing apples of different shapes, sizes and colors as seen in heirloom varieties on old trees. In fact, the US Agricultural Marketing Service has designed a complex system of grading fruit *qualities* by their *appearance*! The current grades are categorized as Extra Fancy, Fancy, Number 1, and Utility. For example, here is what inspectors will look for if you want to market your product as Extra Fancy:

U.S. Extra Fancy - "U.S. Extra Fancy" consists of apples of one variety.. which are mature but not overripe, clean, fairly well formed, free from decay, internal browning, internal breakdown, soft scald, scab, freezing injury, visible water core, and broken skins.. The apples are free from damage caused by bitter pit or Jonathan spot and by smooth solid, slightly rough or rough russeting, or stem or calyx cracks, as well as damage by invisible water core after January 31st of the year following the year of production .. For the apple varieties listed in table 1 of §51.305, each apple of this grade has the amount of color specified for the variety (See §§51.305 and 51.306.)

The problem is that this marketing system is designed to reward factory farms (mechanized, sprayed, gassed) using genetically-modified grades because small biological (regenerative) orchards often do not produce uniform, perfect-looking fruits. Nature's creations are not uniform and perfect the same way humans are not all created of the same size, height and standard complexion, unless we resort to genetic engineering, plastic surgery, chemical cosmetics or Botox!

As usual, in his *quantitative* quest to expand scale, speed and convenience, *Homo economicus* sacrifices and trades away quality. But how can we define the quality of a fruit or food we consume?

In my books, I define quality as "*That which cannot be measured/quantified in the short-term.*" We don't measure the quality of a parent by the size or number of their children, the quality of children by the number of toys or video games they have, or the quality of a friend by his/her perfect appearance. Usually only *time* will judge the quality of anything, particularly when it comes to the health of our body or relationships. For example, a perfect-looking "extra fancy" apple that causes a spike in our blood sugar a few hours after its consumption is of a lower metabolic *quality* (for our body's health) than a small, deformed, tart heirloom variety from a biological (chemical-free) farm, which is digested slowly and therefore, not causing a spike in our blood glucose levels. This is why heirloom varieties like Rhode Island Greening or Newtown Pippin, grown without chemicals in wild nature, in small orchards or someone's backyard may be of better *quality* than pricey Extra Fancy grades. These heirloom varieties are often smaller, more yellow-greenish, tart (acidic sour, less sweet), and have thicker skins, higher density of fiber and vitamins A, B, C, E and K than cross-hybridized perfect looking larger, redder, sweeter, fancier apples.

Facts and Myths about Milk: Does Fat-free Milk Fatten us?

For years, the food industry and their sponsored scientists and regulatory agencies warned people against drinking whole raw milk. Large dairy companies loved the popularity of skim (no-fat) and low-fat milks in the 1980s because that allowed them to separate and churn/turn the most valuable part of the milk, i.e., the creamy fat, containing a good part of vitamin A, D and E, into expensive products like butter and ice cream.

Today, many states still ban the sale of raw milk, while others allow it with a license. Today, practically all packaged milk sold in stores are *homogenized* and *pasteurized*, even if they are still whole-fat and organic. So is there something wrong with milk fat? How about raw milk? Why do dairy companies homogenize, pasteurize and sometimes even *ultra pasteurize* milk? Is fat-free skim milk healthier than whole milk, which contains about 3-4

% fat (depending on the breed of cow and its diet)? Is raw milk safe or unsafe? Are all organic milks the same and worth the extra price we pay for them? Here is a summary of what you may not find on TV or mainstream media. In preparing this summary, I have used research papers as well as my own personal discussions with local farmer friends who run major dairy farms.

Fermented hay (preferably the chemical-free, non-sprayed type) mixed with some alfalfa is cows' favorite food and it helps them make fat-soluble fermented vitamin K2, which together with vitamin D, ensures the calcium in their milk deposits in their baby calves' bones and *not* in their arteries causing *heart attacks*, in joints causing *arthritis*, in kidneys causing kidney stones, or in eyes causing *cataract.* When humans pasteurize the milk at temperatures higher than 150 °F or ultra high temperatures above the boiling point, we mostly *deactivate* the beneficial lactobacilli, the bacteria that facilitate fermentation, as well as vitamins D and K2. In other words, with pasteurization we impair the body's ability to direct calcium into bones and not to unwanted tissues in arteries, kidneys and eyes[11].

The following is a modified excerpt from my book *Masks, Crutches, and Daggers* (on Amazon's 2022 list of Hot New Release):

"Solids and powders may be the preferred form in non-living nature but life forms mostly rely on aqueous (water-based) systems. Milk is one such product. Despite its fat content, milk is mostly water-based. There are natural colloidal forces in the liquid phase between small droplets, like those forces which cause coalescence of milk fat in raw milk into cream, the source of milk's beneficial fat-soluble vitamins A, D, E and K. Again, humans have tried to outsmart (overcome) these natural balancing forces through

---

[11] Adding magnesium, green vegetables and beneficial bacterial products like kefir or sauerkraut to our diet may alleviate some of these risks.

elaborate inventions. For example, when humans decided to live in large dense urban clusters, milk from domesticated cows once supplied fresh and raw to local neighbors became a corporate-traded commodity that had to be transferred, cost-effectively, across long distances to large population centers. The commoditization of fresh milk was in response to, as with other aspects of our new evolutionary path, the simultaneous need for more reach (distance), speed (from cow to factory to warehouse to store shelf to home), convenience (of supermarket vs. driving to a farm) and quantity (large population centers)...

To improve its shelf-life in transit and on stores' refrigerator shelves, raw milk was pasteurized at high temperatures and then homogenized. Apart from the fact that high temperature pasteurization is shown to denature milk proteins and destroy milk's beneficial vitamins and enzymes, the process of homogenization further denatures the milk by breaking up, through force, large fat (cream) globules in the emulsion – liquid in liquid dispersion – from an average diameter of 5 microns to an average of about 0.5 microns. One micron, or micrometer, is one millionth of a meter. This increases the number and surface area of fat (cream) globules by about 1000 times and exposes them to surface oxidation. It is reported that this process not only oxidizes and damages conjugated linoleic acid – a valuable cancer fighting compound in raw milk – but also produces harmful cholesterol oxidation products which are atherogenic – causing formation of fatty plaques in the arteries –, cytotoxic, mutagenic and carcinogenic. In fact, Dr. Kurt Oster's milk studies from the early 1960s until the mid-1980s singled out milk homogenization as a major cause of the current epidemic of heart disease. Although Oster's conclusions are endorsed by the Weston A. Price Foundation, not every researcher agrees with them. Nevertheless, denaturing fresh milk to increase its shelf life as a mass- produced commodity seems to damage some of its key nutrients. As with other decisions we make in our new evolutionary path, we are trading off quality with quantity."

Besides pasteurization and homogenization, industrial dairy farms which buy and distribute milk from farmers, usually separate the purchased milk into its main components of cream (fat), skim (no fat) milk and whey (water soluble proteins). Depending on the percent fat in the final milk or dairy product (like cheese, butter, whey or cream), the *fractionated* (denatured) milk components are mixed back again and packaged into different dairy products. Synthetic vitamins A and D may be added back to low-fat milk because the natural form of these vitamins are lost during the cream removal and heating/pasteurization processes. As a result, packaged milk is a processed (man-made) *denatured* product with controlled fat and added vitamins, and a nutritional profile that is different from that of natural (raw) milk. For example, while whole (raw) milk has a bad reputation because it has more fat than low-fat milk, in reality it is shown that it raises the HDL (good) type cholesterol and improves (reduces) the ratio of Triglycerides to HDL, which is a risk factor with heart disease.

There are also questions about low fat milk leading to weight gain, rather than weight loss. Feeding skim milk or whey to pigs is indeed a technique used by some farmers to quickly fatten their pigs, although feeding them corn or wheat seems even more effective. The effect may be caused by lack of fat (cream) soluble vitamins A,D, E and K and enzymes in skim milk that balance protein and lactose metabolism, hence a faster rise in blood sugar and fat storage in pigs. This may be similar to how humans can gain weight even by eating low-fat food, and related to what I called the 4 Bs of body metabolism earlier.

Here are some other interesting facts about milk:

* Remember it as 3,4,5: Good raw bovine milk contains about 3% protein, 4% fat and 5% lactose (carbohydrate) and the rest is water. Sheep's milk is richer in protein, fat and lactose and less watery.

* Bovine milk protein is 80% casein (larger water insoluble proteins that curdle into cheese by cultures or into yogurt by lactic acid bacteria) and 20% whey (smaller water soluble protein molecules) but human milk is 30% casein and 70% whey so cow's milk is not an ideal metabolic replacement for human milk. On a related note, whey protein powders are isolated (denatured) and also difficult to metabolize for humans.

* Some nutritionists believe that the natural proteins, enzymes and hormones in cow's milk cause metabolic, digestive and hormonal disruptions, abnormal growth but also risk of cancer, lactose intolerance, excessive mucosal activity and immune response, and even autoimmune diseases in some humans. Other nutritionists blame these not on all cows but on hormone-fed vaccinated and medicated cows raised in commercial caged factory farms on non-organic (sprayed) grains, hay or grass. I am not an expert on these matters. Perhaps one can test their sensitivities by trying high quality milk in their diet or better yet, ferment it to products like yogurt or kefir to break down many of the questionable proteins and sugars (lactose) and make them more digestible and compatible with our body. Similar to animal proteins, proteins, hormones and growth factors in cow's milk may artificially boost the anabolic cellular growth pathways both in healthy and cancerous cells.

* Raw milk can be sterilized at around 150 °F. Yet, despite its increasing popularity, sale of raw milk is banned in many states and countries under pressure by the commercial milk industry. As a result, small dairy farmers can not directly sell their products so many are going out of business. There is also a lot of pressure on the mass media not to discuss raw milk. For example, an article in the Supermarket News titled "Australia is in a raw market frenzy" was removed after publication.

* The deeper the yellowness or orange tint of the cream in raw whole milk, the more β-carotene (vitamin A precursor) it contains, usually indicating the cow was free ranging on grasslands, in contrast to caged corn- or alfalfa-fed cows. The main carotenoids identified in grass foragers are lutein, β-carotene, and zeaxanthin. Certain breeds like the Guernsey and Jersey cattle produce less milk but more golden cream containing more beta carotene per day than breeds like Holsteins.

Eye-Opening Facts About Eggs and Chickens

Not all eggs are created equal. A 2021 study by Shuangshi Wei et al. shows the efficacy of egg yolk antibodies (IgY) as a neutralizing agent against SARS-CoV-2 in protecting people against symptomatic COVID-19. Humans have long used eggs as a nutritious and healing food. But unfortunately, much of the eggs in the market today are mass-produced. Following are some facts about the egg industry definitions (organic, cage-free, free-range, pasture- raised, etc.) you will most likely not hear on your TV, in mass media or from most celebrities ("attention merchants") because many of them are sponsored by food companies and don't work for us.

For starters, certain breeds of chickens like Bovans Brown have been selectively cross-bred, hybridized and *denatured* by humans to unnaturally produce more than 300 eggs a year at the expense of their shorter lifespans of about 2-3 years, in contrast to their natural cousins like Ruffed Grouse and Prairie chickens that can live 8-12 years. Chicks of the denatured egg-laying breeds are often machine-incubated and machine-hatched in large commercial hatcheries, in contrast to natural chicks slowly hatching under a brooding caring mother chicken. Commercial incubated eggs are then delivered by large food companies in truckloads to egg farms, which are often contractors to large food companies. But most egg farms are *not* farms and are just large walled structures ventilated and temperature-controlled to make sure chickens stay alive. Trust me. Those charming rustic pastoral images you see on egg cartons are not what an egg factory looks like! Many egg farms pack 10,000-50,000 layer chickens in compact shelved areas that provide only 1-2 square feet of space per chicken. Caged layers (Egg-laying chickens), unlike free chickens that pick/peck their food from pastures, are fed *processed* food. Today, many *cage-free* facilities are actually multiple-story structures like one recently built in Iowa that crams 540,000 chickens inside.

After about a year of producing about an egg a day, these boxed and often vaccinated and medicated chickens become hard to control. Because chickens explore the world with their beaks, if there isn't adequate space in their environment, they won't have enough ground space to peck, thus leading them to peck on each other. Not only can this cause infections if a bird is preening her feathers or pecks at an insect on a flock-mate that leads to minor skin wounds, but it can also eventually lead to cannibalism and aggression. In addition, too little space for chickens means quick accumulation of manure and droppings, repulsive stench and poor quality breathing air despite some ventilation. So after about 12 months of laying numerous eggs, traumatized exhausted chickens are often taken to a slaughterhouse for their meat[12] before they die of extreme sickness. Chickens generate a lot of profits for humans while living a tortured life.

So by now, you may have an idea why it is wise to raise your own eggs or buy from farms that do not overstress their chickens. Happy pasture-raised chickens roam free range on grassland, protected by a rooster

---

[12] Broiler (meat/broiler) chickens don't even grow old enough to lay eggs and are fattened to about six pounds in six weeks and slaughtered then.

from hawks, foxes and raccoons. When we treat our chickens right, their eggs will treat us well.

Contrary to a public misconception, the color of the egg shell is *not* correlated with its nutrient density or value so brown colored eggs are not necessarily more nutritious than white eggs! The nutritional quality of an egg is a function of the diet and health of the chicken laying it, which in turn depends on how naturally the chicken was born and raised. Generally-speaking, the pigments that determine the egg shell's colors are also present in chicken's skin, legs, and earlobes. Other factors that may affect egg color are age, season and even diet. In commercial farming, where hens are fed a diet of corn and soy, the eggs are more likely to be white. Apart from natural variations, store-bought eggs may come in unnatural colors as well. This is due to the commercial egg production industry adding feed additives that can change the color of the eggshell.

Unfortunately, there are also a lot of labeling gimmicks in the egg market. Beware of some eggs marketed as organic or cage-free because "organic" could mean organic *grain-fed* but not entirely pasture-raised. "Cage-free" or "free-range" could mean large congested holding areas. The government does not have any requirements around what the outdoor environment should be like, or how much time chickens get to spend outdoors. In California, an enclosure containing nine or more egg-laying hens shall provide a minimum of about 0.8 square feet of floor space per bird. Most other states do not even have such a requirement. Here are some industry terms and definitions:

"Caged": Hens are confined to cages with a 67-square inch space each. They never see the light of day and consume a corn or soy diet. The egg carton will often not say caged and may even have a nice picture of a barn or a farm. Over 90% of eggs in the U.S. come from hens that are kept in cages for their entire egg-laying lives[13] (further explained below).

"Cage-Free": These hens have more room than caged hens but still less than 1 square foot! So they're not really "free," since they're confined to barns and consume a corn or soy diet.

"Free-Range": Allotted less than 2 square feet per hen, these animals have more space than their caged and cage-free peers, but they don't get outdoors as much as you may think. Some seldom get to see the light of day and many still eat a corn- or soy-based feed.

"Pasture-Raised": These ladies are given at least 108 square feet each and consume some feed and lots of grass, bugs, worms and anything else they can find in the dirt. They tend to be let out of the barns early in the morning and called back in before nightfall. You may have to pay 2-3 times more for pasture-raised eggs than for other types of eggs. According to a 2003 study out of Pennsylvania State University one pasture-raised egg contains twice as much omega-3 fat, three times more vitamin D, four times more vitamin E and seven times more beta-carotene (the yolk's orangish color) than cheaper store-bought eggs.

Here are other interesting facts[14] about chickens:

At any given time, there are about 300 million egg-laying hens on farms in the U.S. A majority of these birds are kept in battery cages—small enclosures where several birds are crammed in. Caged birds suffer from poor living conditions—they have no room to move around, their stress levels are very high and, not surprisingly, they are aggressive toward each other. Cages are filthy, increasing the risk of bacterial infections and necessitating the use of antibiotics (which is bad practice when done on a precautionary basis rather than to treat an existing infection). Caged chickens, by

---

[13] https://certifiedhumane.org/

[14] www.diffen.com/difference/Caged_Chicken_vs_Free_Range_Chicken

definition, have almost no opportunity to live naturally, and sometimes share their cages with dead chickens. Caged chickens are usually kept in battery cages their entire productive life; they can barely stand up, cannot spread their wings, and are denied natural behaviors like roosting, nesting, perching and bathing.

Cage-free birds live in aviaries large enough to hold thousands of birds. These are industrial barns where there is about 1 square foot of space available per hen. A research study by the Coalition for Sustainable Egg Supply found that benefits of cage-free aviaries for the birds include more natural behavior, stronger bones and more feathers. But cage-free birds also face risks—mortality rate is much higher (slightly more than 10%) than caged birds (about 5%) because of pecking by other birds. And without access to the outdoors, the quality of indoor air in aviaries can be poor.

Free-range in theory means cage-free with access to the outdoors. However, there is no other requirement around this access. While free-range chickens have some opportunity to experience natural behaviors, how much opportunity is entirely unregulated and unmonitored. In fact, a majority of free-range birds actually do not venture outdoors because the outdoor environment is often simply a fenced porch with little to no grass, bushes or worms. So in practice, free-range and cage-free provide the same living conditions.

Pasture-raised chickens have the best living conditions among poultry farms today. They are not confined in cages or aviaries, spending most of their time outdoors where they have access to a natural diet of insects and worms ....

What chickens eat and how much they are treated with hormones and antibiotics are the largest factors in the nutritional value, flavor, and even safety for human consumption of their eggs and meat. While there are no organizations monitoring the validity of caged and free-range chicken nutrition, the assumptions can be made that Grain-fed chickens will grow faster and fatter than pasture-raised chickens.

The Quality of Meat from Factory Farms

There are more than 20,000 concentrated animal feeding operations (CAFOs) in the U.S.. These refer to intensive animal feeding operations in which over 700 dairy cows, or 1,000 meat cows or 10,000 pigs weighing under 55 pounds or 10,000 sheep or 55,000 turkeys or 125,000 chickens, or 82,000 egg laying hens or pullets are confined for over 45 days a year. These operations that produce much of the meat people consume in America are extremely stressful for the animals and also generate tons of manure which poses substantial risks to the water and air quality and public health. If you ever visit any of these facilities up close you would probably stop eating any meat raised in such operations. Cameras and reporters are usually not allowed in these facilities but movies and documentaries like *Fast Food Nation* and *Food, Inc.* have portrayed the problems associated with such facilities.

Most people may not realize that the high stress levels experienced by maltreated animals in factory farms, besides making them prone to all sorts of diseases, will impact their meat too.

After unstressed or low-stress animals die in the wild, their muscle glycogen is converted anaerobically – which means in the absence of oxygen, because oxygenated blood is no longer flowing – into lactic acid. This is the acid that keeps meat tender, pink, flavorful and resistant to harmful bacteria. When animals are stressed, however, like when they are kept in packed, smelly and hot factory farms and transported to crowded slaughter stations while hearing other animals moan in fear, their body and muscles release stress hormones adrenaline and cortisol. These hormones use up glycogen (energy) storage in muscles, which means less lactic acid will be formed. Such meat will be darker, drier, tougher, less acidic and therefore more susceptible to microbial contamination. Much of the meat in supermarkets is kept *artificially* red and denatured by packing it in artificial atmospheres like

80% oxygen and 20% carbon dioxide. This technique is called Modified Atmosphere Packaging (MAP).

I personally believe the abundance of stress hormones in the stressed animal meat would also negatively impact the hormonal balance of people consuming such meat.

Chapter 4: Pesticides and GMOs in Food

Today, the bulk of food sold in stores are from sources that have been sprayed with synthetic petroleum-based chemical pesticides, including fruits, vegetables, grains, and feedstock for the meat we consume. Many grains and fruits are also genetically modified organisms (GMOs). I would avoid whenever possible foods from sprayed sources especially in vegetables and fruits which could be consumed raw. The "Dirty Dozen" list, updated annually by the EWG (The Environmental Working Group), outlines which produce items are most likely to contain pesticides. Their list includes strawberries, apples, nectarines, peaches, celery, grapes, cherries, spinach, tomatoes, sweet bell peppers, cherry tomatoes and cucumbers. Generally, fruits and vegetables with high water and sugar contents, and thinner skins are vulnerable. Seeds and nuts like almond and walnut are also heavily sprayed and/or fumigated with chemicals after harvest.

The following is an overview of the scientific literature about pesticides and whether they impact fertility, masculinity and miscarriages.

In 1962, Rachel Carson's best-seller *Silent Spring* warned the world that pesticides, which were marketed, for the most part deceptively, to farmers after World War II, act like toxic nerve agents and wreak havoc on our bodies, our planet and its animals, particularly fragile birds and fish. In the U.S., entire cities like Detroit – from the air! – and groups, like children in Texas, were regularly sprayed with pesticides. By 1980's nearly all persons tested had pesticide compounds in their blood. Although Carson's book led to the banning of DDT, and books like *Toxic Legacy: How the Weedkiller Glyphosate Is Destroying Our Health and the Environment* by scientist Stephanie Seneff have shared more recent compelling evidence against pesticides, humans are using pesticides more than ever before, currently at a rate of one pound per year for each living person on the planet. Between 1990 and 2020, average pesticide usage worldwide increased by 50%. This Chapter reviews trusted scientific evidence from countries across the world about reproductive and neurological harms associated with pesticides.

Nerve Agents Sprayed onto Farms?

Synthetic petroleum-based pesticides are designed to eradicate weeds, insects and fungi that reduce crop yields in non-organic farming. Genetically-modified crops either integrate the pesticide chemistry into the crop seeds or ensure when they are sprayed they can resist the pesticide (glyphosate for example so they call it glyphosate-ready) and not wither or die. There are two major types of chemistries used as pesticides:

Organochlorine pesticides such as DDT, Atrazine (of Triazine class), and 2,4-D[15] (a component of the notorious chemical weapon called "Agent Orange") are chemically stable and strongly fat-loving – lipophilic – so their residues not degraded or excreted from the body tend to "bioaccumulate" in lipid-rich (fatty) tissues in the body such as in the brain and our nervous system in the fatty myelin sheath covering neurons. These compounds have also received the most attention because of their persistence in the environment, their ability to concentrate up the food web, and their continuous detection in the food supply and drinking water. They also seem to accumulate in organisms and then can cause endocrine (hormonal) disruption (explained further below).

Organophosphorus (OP) pesticides such as glyphosate and malathion use phosphorus chemistry (instead of chlorine) which is also used in insecticides,

---

[15] DICHLORO:diphenyltrichloroethane=DDT; phenoxyacetic acid=2,4D

herbicides, nerve gas or nerve agents like Sarin in chemical warfare, and in low cost flame-retardants in fabrics and furniture. Some organophosphates are potent nerve agents, functioning by inhibiting the action of an enzyme[16] in our nervous system which activates and balances our motor neurons and muscles. So pesticides, fire retardants and certain venoms (produced by plants and snakes), which result in accumulation of acetylcholine cause continuous stimulation of the muscles, glands, and central nervous system and may lead to fatal convulsions, muscular paralysis, bronchial constriction, death by asphyxiation as well as brain disorders such as memory loss, foggy brain, Alzheimer's disease, depression, irritability, confusion and sleep disorders.

In bees and certain other animals and insects, exposure to organophosphorus insecticides and chlorinated hydrocarbons are associated with aggressiveness, paralysis and abnormal activities, as explained in a paper by D.F. Mayer. The most common symptoms of bee poisoning are the appearance of dead bees in front of the hives, abnormal communication dances and disorganized behavior, infertility of the queen, and regurgitation of the honey stomach. According to the National Caucus of Environmental Legislators, exposure to organophosphates often disrupts the bees' ability to find pollen and return to the hive, leaving the colony vulnerable to developing colony collapse disorder. Foragers returning to the hive with a load of contaminated pollen or nectar can cause extreme agitation and death of other bees.

Organophosphate pesticides can be absorbed by humans through inhalation, ingestion, and dermal (skin)

---

[16] Acetylcholinesterase (AChE) which helps break down acetylcholine (ACh), the neurotransmitter controlling our muscle tones and movements.

absorption. Their toxicity is not limited to the acute phase, however, and chronic long-term effects such as foggy brain have long been noted. Neurotransmitters such as acetylcholine which are affected by organophosphate pesticides are profoundly important in the brain's development, so many organophosphates have neurotoxic effects on developing organisms, even from low levels of exposure. Fetuses and young children, whose brain development depends on a strict sequence of biological events, may be most at risk, according to *Everyday Environmental Toxins* edited by Areej Hassan.

In most of the studies conducted in North America, glyphosate and atrazine are the two commonly found pesticides in water bodies.

Infertility, Miscarriages and Birth Defects

Certain chemicals in plastics and pesticides are structurally so similar to our hormones (like estrogens) that they may confuse our body and cause disruptions in our endocrine (hormonal) systems especially the female hormone estrogen. The estrogenic effects of endocrine-disrupting chemicals found in pesticides have also been well characterized in a number of assay systems, leading to the conclusion that many pesticides adversely affect *reproductive* outcomes, by causing *birth defects, pregnancy complications or infertility.* Many pesticides are known to cross the human placenta, and these compounds can be found in the tissues of mothers and newborns. In a cohort of 325 women undergoing infertility treatment with assisted reproductive technology, studied by Yu-Han Chiu, intake of high–pesticide residue fruits and vegetables was associated with a lower probability of live birth.

In Argentina, maternal residential proximity to rural fruit croplands with intense pesticide applications was associated in a study by Amalia Cecchi with pregnancy complications and alterations in their newborn parameters.

In Iran, a study by Mojtaba Abbasi-Jorjandi confirms severe oxidative stress caused by both organophosphorus and organochlorine Pesticides in the families of farmworkers.

In Ecuador, organophosphates were linked in a paper by Jose Suarez-Lopez to increased depression and anxiety, particularly among women.

Different animal models of exposure to glyphosate or glyphosate-based herbicides have shown that the effects on the female reproductive tract may be related to an "endocrine-disruption" effect. Studies have also demonstrated that the exposure to glyphosate-based herbicides can harm both fertility (by altering the development of ovarian follicles and uterus) and birth defects (by altering the development of the offspring during gestation).

Researchers like Rahul Pathak who studied the risk of abortions and miscarriages found associations with exposure to pesticides and smoking. In Northern India, a study suggests that high blood levels of a chemical found in Lindane, a broad-spectrum chlorinated pesticide, may be associated with risk of recurrent pregnancy loss.

Exposure to endocrine-disrupting chemicals in pesticides prenatally (before birth) or during adult life can have a transgenerational effect on the reproductive health of "future generations" as stated by researchers Emily Brehm and Jodi A Flaws.

Pesticides may also be harmful for reproductive health in *men*. For example, research by Barbara A Cohn confirms that a woman's exposure to DDT increases her son's risk of testicular cancer up to 30 years later! Also, epidemiological research and animal models studied by Philippa D. Darbre strongly link several male reproductive health problems prevalent in Western countries, including hypospadias (abnormal opening of urethra in penis) and cryptorchidism (urogenital tract malformations), abnormalities of spermatogenesis (declining sperm counts and sperm quality), alterations to puberty, development of prostatic hyperplasia (abnormal enlargement), and gynecomastia (man breasts or inappropriate male breast growth) with exposure to estrogenic chemicals and endocrine disruptors such as those found in pesticides, plastics and additives.

Research has also confirmed that certain pesticides such as Vinclozolin (a fungicide) are known antiandrogens and can affect reproduction in male rats by altering sperm function.

Gender Identification and Transgenderism

Pesticides could also interfere with gender identification. Transgender or gender dysphoria is defined in the fifth edition of the Diagnostic and Statistical Manual of Mental Disorders (DSM-5), as "*The incongruence between one's experienced gender and one's assigned gender, along with a persistent and strong desire to be of another gender, and accompanied by clinically significant distress.*" Transsexualism involves prenatal neuroanatomical changes, has a psychiatric association, and is found by researchers like Philippa D. Darbre to be more prevalent in conjunction with schizophrenia. Endocrine disruptors like those in plastics, synthetic perfumes, and pesticides, may be the cause of high fetal testosterone exposure leading to increased risk of autism spectrum disorders as well as gender dysphoria.

Atrazine, for example, is shown to induce complete feminization and chemical castration in male African frogs. The 2010 study by Hayes et. al examined sex ratios, testosterone levels, sexual dimorphism, reproductive behaviors, and fertility in 40 genetically male frogs exposed to 2.5 ppb (parts per billion) atrazine throughout the larval period and for up to 3 years after metamorphosis. The study showed that 10% of the atrazine-exposed animals were chromosomal males which turned into females (lacked visible nuptial pads on the forearms and had protruding cloacal labia and ovaries typical of females) and produced viable eggs. Atrazine exposure also resulted in a significant reduction in the relative number of testicular tubules in about 45% of the tested animals. Also, among the atrazine-treated males which did not feminize, only two out-competed control (untreated natural) males in mating with females and egg fertilization. In addition, Atrazine-treated males, even those with relatively high sperm content, had significantly lower fertility rates and proportions of eggs fertilized, vs. natural frogs.

The results of the frog study are also consistent with other studies that examined long-term behavioral effects of atrazine in fish. Salmon exposed to atrazine (≥6 ppb) showed a dose-dependent decrease in androgens, sperm production and the ability to respond to the attractant female pheromone.

Atrazine exposure is highly correlated in a study by Shanna H Swan with demasculinization of rodents and with low sperm count, poor semen quality, and impaired fertility in male humans. Unfortunately, Atrazine has been widely applied to eliminate broadleaved weeds and perennial grasses in U.S. corn fields since the early 1960s. Globally, it is popularly used on corn as well as pineapples, sugarcane and many other crops. Atrazine has been banned for use in the European Union because of its established pathology.

Other Diseases and Disorders

According to IARC (International Agency for Research on Cancer) *Monographs 112 on the Evaluation of Carcinogenic Risks to Humans*, because of the lipophilic (fat-loving) nature of synthetic (petroleum-based) pesticides, exposure to them affects primarily the nervous system, liver, bone marrow and the brain. Pesticide exposure has been associated by EPA (Environmental Protection Agency) to cancers of liver, prostate, kidney and blood (leukemia) and to neurological disorders in the brain such as Parkinson's disease.

A recent study by Kimberly C. Paul, published in *Nature*, associates long-term exposure to 53 pesticides with Parkinson's disease as a result of toxicity to dopaminergic neurons and mitochondrial dysfunction. About one fourth of epidemiologically implicated pesticides tested in vitro resulted in substantial dopaminergic neuron cell death.

Due to their endocrine-disrupting nature, many pesticides disrupt not only our reproductive system but also our thyroid and adrenal functions, leading to adverse outcomes such as unexplained obesity and weight gain, sweating, feeling too hot or too cold, mood instability, fatigue and excessive inflammation as a result of adrenal fatigue (explained further in *The Rogue Brain*), and unhealthy hair, skin and nails. Pesticides could also impact our gut microbiome and lead to food sensitivities, brain fog, digestive problems and allergies and auto-immune disorders.

Pesticides also adversely impact reproductive health and immune status of farm animals like sheep and cows according to a study by Torres Sweeney. In Uganda, according to a paper by Sabrina Krief, 25% of monitored wild chimpanzees in forests, which raided nearby pesticide-sprayed corn farms (with glyphosate, chlorpyrifos, 2,4-D and others) exhibited abnormalities like reduced nostrils, cleft lip, limb deformities, reproductive problems and hypopigmentation.

The Economics of Pesticides and GMO Seeds

There is a lot of evidence, including those published by the Union of Concerned Scientists, that weeds and insects develop resistance over time to pesticides. Genetically-engineered (GE) seeds, which I prefer to call "genetically-adulterated" or altered, came onto the US agricultural scene in the late 1990s when corporate scientists engineered seeds for plants that could withstand the spraying of the herbicide glyphosate, allowing farmers to spray over growing corn while killing weeds. For about three years (1996-1999) GE seeds achieved what they promised which is increasing yield while decreasing the amount of pesticides applied. But soon that changed and glyphosate-tolerant soybeans and corn needed more weed killers than their non-GE neighbors because weeds evolved resistance and immunity to the chemicals, as reported by Dan Charles for NPR.

Other seeds have been engineered to produce their own insecticide (known as Bacillus thuringiensis or Bt), with the hopes of limiting insecticide spraying. For a while, adopters of insect-resistant engineered maize used less insecticide than nonadopters but there is now evidence that insects such as corn rootworms have evolved resistance to one of the genes that has been deployed against them in Bt corn. This means a constant line of new products and profits for the corporations and higher costs for farmers.

Although yield in organic (non sprayed) farms can be up to 25% less than conventional sprayed farms – except in crops like rye, hay, alfalfa, safflower and oats that organic seem to do well – analysis of USDA survey data shows that operating, and operating plus capital costs per acre for crop production are generally less for organic than for conventional farms which have significantly higher seed, fertilizer, and chemical costs but lower labor costs.

So the higher yields achieved by using synthetic petroleum-based pesticides (whether sprayed or genetically integrated into engineered seeds) or GMO seeds are both transient and costly. They lead in the long term to pesticide resistance as well as disastrous ecological, neurological and reproductive problems.

Soil, Water and Gut Health

Pesticide applications are often inefficient and associated with reduction in soil fertility and microbiome diversity. There are concerns for the persistence of pesticides in both surface and ground waters (as documented in the book *Toxic Deception*) and even in rainwater. Some 30–50% of the applied pesticides may also end up on the soil surface according to a study by Sajjad Ali. Such pesticide-contaminated soil particles, carried up to the atmosphere with the wind, make rainwater infertile for Vitamin B12 because the soil is often devoid of any living microorganisms. If you recall from Chapter 2, certain soil microbes are essential for synthesizing vitamin B12, whether on the ground, in our guts or inside rain droplets.

Studies such as those by Florian Walder have also consistently reported long-term adverse effects of pesticides on the soil nitrogen cycle (soil fertility), and transient adverse effects on abundance, diversity or composition of soil microbial communities. In fact, pesticide residues were negatively associated (harmful) with bacterial diversity but positively with fungal diversity. This is perhaps linked to fungi's capability to produce enzymes to biodegrade pesticides. Pesticides can affect the competition for ecological niches by giving advantages to pesticide-resistant microbes. Overall, pesticides seem to drastically disturb the natural microbial balance and health of the soil as well as the food that grows in it (grains, vegetables and animal feedstock). Pesticide residues remaining on food make their way into our digestive tract and disrupt the functioning of beneficial bacteria in our guts and contribute to inflammatory and autoimmune disorders such as Celiac disease and certain cancers.

Chapter 5: How Does Bad Food Make Us Sick?

In Chapter 2, I discussed our body's telltale signs of imbalance caused by bad food choices. Here I will describe how bad food can cause or aggravate diseases.

Bad food contains ingredients that disrupt our metabolism and energy balance starting at the cellular level. Mitochondria are organelles inside our cells that convert glucose and fat in our food and oxygen from the air, all delivered in the bloodstream, to renewable energy storage packets that are exchanged inside the body as our energy currency. These molecules (called ATP) are like rechargeable batteries that keep recharging inside our mitochondria and across our body. All our cells, including our muscles (heart and limbs) and neurons inside our brain and our peripheral nervous system rely on the energy produced in this process to function properly and with vitality.

Yet, there are many denatured forces and chemicals that are "mitochondrial disruptors" and can interact with and disrupt the process inside mitochondria (called electron transport chain). These include energy waves (like 5G signals from microwaves and cell phones) that can disrupt calcium signaling in the body, as well as any denatured (processed) chemicals in their metastable energy states in our food, water, air, toothpastes, shampoos, deodorants, medicines, etc. The long list includes elements such as mercury, lead, aluminum, iron, fluoride, chlorine, synthetic compounds like pesticides, medicines (like metformin, statins, pain killer, etc.), denatured fats like seed oils containing omega 6 and metastable fatty acids prone to oxidation, alcohol, synthetic food additives and dyes, toxins, infections and basically anything that creates oxidative stress and loss of electrons. Dr. Peter Rogers has a series of educational videos on Youtube about this topic. Although I may not agree with *all* his dietary conclusions (he avoids all meat and fat), I find his videos sincere and educational.

Certain substances like caffeine, melatonin (sleep), meat proteins, selenium and vitamins B and C could actually stimulate the electron transfer chain but deplete magnesium which ATP needs to become biologically active. That is why coffee drinkers, meat eaters and people using vitamin supplements need extra magnesium found in green leaves and vegetables in their diet. Most vegetables in their natural state contain the proper balance of vitamins and magnesium anyway.

So what happens when we disrupt the electron transport chain inside our cellular power plants? In some cases, out-of-control oxidative chain reactions happen which not only impair our energy level but also damage our cells and our DNA, which is equivalent to aging. In such cases of metabolic dysfunction, our wounds would not heal quickly, we would get sick easily and remain sick longer. We would experience pain, brain fog or headache. Basically our immune system would not have enough resources to protect or repair us in an efficient manner.

Fruits and vegetables (of low denaturation score) high in vitamin C, magnesium and micronutrients like polyphenol could help with restoration of our cellular energy. But the best strategy is to avoid any food, water or consumables (like toothpastes with fluoride or deodorants with aluminum compounds) that can disrupt our cellular metabolism. We now have enough evidence to link several physical and neurological diseases such as dementia and Alzheimer's to mitochondrial disruptors in our food, water and air.

A major problem with mitochondrial disruptions, prolonged oxidative stress inside our cells and out-of-control reactions consuming oxygen is the increased risk of <u>cancer</u>. This state of hypoxia (oxygen deficiency) can lead to cancer according to polymath and Nobel laureate Otto Warburg. He showed that cancer is an extreme survival mechanism by our cells when they are choking (hypoxic) and suffer from a throttled mitochondrial metabolism. These *denatured* cells switch from aerobic to anaerobic (oxygen-starved) glycolysis (metabolism of glucose). Certain carcinogenic factors that could cause this dangerous mutation in our body include sugar, chemicals in pesticides, medicines and drugs, artificial food additives, electromagnetic radiation, chronic stressors and other factors that deprive our body of adequate oxygen such as smoking (or even long-term use of face masks?), high blood pressure, clogged arteries, etc.

Apart from wreaking havoc on our cellular energy factories, bad food disrupts other processes in our body such as our digestion. We already mentioned how denatured foods concentrated in sugar and sodium salt can cause diabetes and hypertension (high blood pressure), respectively, and how petroleum-derived pesticides or food additives can disrupt our nervous system functions and gut bacteria. Basically, any food ingredient that unnaturally or excessively triggers our body's burn, build, break down or bury could lead to disease. In *The Rogue Brain* I explain how disease is basically a state of severe *metabolic imbalance* or allostatic load in our body. For example, many molecules in synthetic plastics, pesticides, vaccines, medicine and denatured processed food could trigger autoimmune diseases and hormonal imbalances because the synthetic molecules chemically resemble our body's endogenous natural proteins or hormones, which are metabolic or immune signaling molecules.

Chapter 6: The 10 Commandments of Eating

As we approach the end of this book, I would like to suggest my 10 commandments of eating well, which I try to faithfully follow:

1- Do Not Eat or Use Denatured Food! Especially any food with a denaturation score worse than -8. Ideally use raw natural food like chemical-free potato, garlic, carrots, barley, etc. Other examples of denatured foods are seedless fruits like seedless melons and grapes, concentrated powders like sugar or bleached flour, concentrated drinks like orange juice and alcohol. Coffee is mostly a denatured food and can denature your metabolism if not consumed with enough greens and magnesium. In moderation, however, it can boost our vigilance, attention, metabolism and energy when we are fatigued. Like all concentrated and refined food, however, coffee is strongly addictive so it can become a *crutch* that should be avoided or minimized.

2- Farm or Know your Farmer! When the farmers who grow your food, the soil they use, and the animals they raise are stressed and imbalanced, your food is imbalanced and of low quality. Try to learn and spend the time to grow your food or at least a part of it or buy as much of it as possible fresh and in season from small chemical-free farms. Mass-produced commodity food is optimized for shelf life, quantity, appearance and cost, and usually not for quality and metabolic wholesomeness.

3- Balance Your Plate! Most denatured food today is imbalanced and deficient in some essential nutrients. If you are not buying or producing natural wholesome foods, you need to balance any excess in calcium with magnesium in greens, dehydrated food with water, sodium with potassium (in vegetables like potatoes), sugars, proteins and fats with fiber (from vegetables) and probiotic bacteria from fermented foods (like sauerkraut or kefir). It's good to also balance food groups against each other. For example meats with vegetables, herbs and fermented foods, or starches with fats and vegetables. Some nutritionists recommend a colorfully-balanced rainbow palette on your plate, like balancing red tomatoes with green lettuce and orange sweet potatoes because as discussed earlier, the color of micronutrients may be an indicator of their position on the metabolic spectrum.

4- Do Not Eat Until You Feel the "Real" Hunger! Please review chapters 1 and 2 or *The Rogue Brain* on how to stop your stressed or addicted brain to impose "fake hunger" and bad food on you, which leads to numerous health issues.

5- Be Regular! Regularity in food, sleep and poop cycles will reduce metabolic stresses on your body especially if your cycles follow your body's natural circadian hormonal patterns. For example, the catabolic hormone cortisol that breaks down fat and glycogen energy reserves into glucose naturally dips after sunset and peaks around sunrise in anticipation of our energy needs. If we stay up late, are active later in the day, or eat heavy meals after sunset, we disrupt our body's natural circadian cortisol pattern and energy management strategy. Caffeine drinks such as coffee act like artificial cortisol, temporarily boosting our energy and attention. But if consumed more than a cup or anytime after noon, they will disrupt our cortisol functionality and natural energy flow. In fact, flat cortisol patterns that are too low or too high throughout the day have been associated with major depressive disorders.

6- Eat Slow and in Peace, Savor the Flavor in Good Food! During our meals, nothing can help our digestive and metabolic processes more than peace. Avoid thoughts, talks, or people involving money and time (deadlines)! Savor your food peacefully in nature or in the fellowship of peaceful grateful people you trust. Chew well with your mouth closed.

7- Avoid Artificial Additives, GMO and Sprayed Food! Many artificial additives and colors (like Red 40) in food and chemicals in pesticides are linked to neurological disorders, migraine headaches, brain fog, and are banned in Europe. Avoid colored food unless colored naturally (like by turmeric or beet juice).

8- Minimize or Stop Packaged Food! Plastics can leach chemicals, including hormone disruptors, especially when warm, exposed to liquids and acidic food, or microwaved. Try to avoid water and liquid food packaged in plastic, metal or paper packages (which are usually plastic-coated and hot-filled). Glass is usually the best choice for packaging. Don't drink your hot drinks or foods in foam or plastic containers. Ceramic and glass containers are much better choices.

9- Cook Your Food at Home but Don't Microwave! Cooking food on gas stoves in stainless or ceramic coated pots and pans is OK. Aluminum and teflon-coated cookware are linked to health problems. Cast iron, if seasoned not to leach, is occasionally OK. Spending the time to prepare and cook good food is the best investment in your health because you will use only quality and balanced ingredients, and prepare it with love and caring, and not for profit. Much of restaurant and packaged foods are mass-produced by unhappy workers, with low quality imbalanced (denatured) ingredients, not fresh, and high in sugar, additives, sodium salts and fat.

10- Limit Your Meat Consumption! Unless your job or athletic activity requires heavy muscular work, or you are a teenager or a muscularly-weak elderly person in need of muscle growth or retention, *limiting* meat in your daily diet is probably a good idea, especially factory meats, chicken and pork.

Chapter 7: On Gluten, Detox and Supplements

Food is often a perplexing topic because humans still do not fully understand: (1) How does modifying the food source to increase its yield by techniques like seed selection, hybridization and gene-editing (as in GMO seeds) impact the biochemical composition and bioavailability of ingredients in new human-altered foods?; and (2) How does the human body metabolize these genetically-altered foods or other modern foods processed with all the additives?

For example, the topic of gluten and gluten-resistance, or lactose and lactose-intolerance have been debated for years. Is gluten the real culprit for many of our gut and health issues like autoimmune conditions? These discussions are beyond the scope of this book and my expertise. I believe we still do not have answers to many of our food-related questions. But here I will try to share my views about some of these controversies.

Gluten

Gluten is a protein naturally found in certain grains such as wheat, barley, and rye, which acts like a binder and forms an elastic "stretchable" network. This is what makes bread and pizza doughs stretchable. Bread and pizza flours are higher than pastry and all-purpose flours in gluten content. Rice, buckwheat, corn, quinoa, oats and certain types of wheat like einkorn have little or no gluten. Sourdough breads also have lower levels of gluten because the slow fermentation process allows yeast and bacteria to break down some of the gluten. We often make our own sourdough fresh at home by grinding small batches of whole grain chemical-free local grains, mix half and half with organic unbleached bread flour, and use fermentation starters like kefir or yogurt. There are many easy methods to do this, which you can find online, but like all other good things in life all these methods need *time and patience.*

Gluten has been blamed for adverse, inflammatory, immunological, and autoimmune reactions in about 1% of the population suffering from celiac disease, which is an autoimmune disorder causing fatigue, bloating, alternating constipation and diarrhea, unintentional weight loss, malnutrition and intestinal damage.

Because removing the gluten from whole grains denatures them, it is not advisable for non-celiac individuals. Consuming wholesome whole grains has been associated with significantly lower rates of heart disease and stroke, type 2 diabetes, and deaths from all causes[17]. Gluten is also a prebiotic, which means it feeds the "good" bacteria in our gut, of course if our food ingredients are not sprayed with pesticides!

So, is gluten really to blame for triggering celiac disease in certain people? Some people believe it is the abnormally high gluten and protein content of denatured modern wheat varieties that is causing the issue. Analyses have shown that gluten content has remained constant over the last 120 years[18], although higher rain precipitation in the year of the harvest was accompanied by a higher gluten content in the samples. So, could it be commercial farming and unnatural irrigation practices that have impacted gluten content in modern wheat varieties?

Another factor that may have changed in recent years is the content of Amylase Trypsin Inhibitor (ATI), which wheat plants produce as a natural pesticide to protect themselves from insects. A few generations ago, wheat breeders began to select for higher insect resistance, which has resulted in ATI levels in modern wheat cultivars that are much higher than heirloom varieties. ATI is known as a major wheat allergen and it is possible

---

[17] https://nutritionsource.hsph.harvard.edu/gluten/
[18] https://www.sciencedaily.com/releases/2020/08/200811120112.htm

that Celiac disease actually starts as an allergy to the ATI in wheat flour and evolves into an inability of the intestines to handle gluten[19].

A third potential cause of wheat allergies is the use of synthetic pesticides on the majority of non-organic wheat in the United States treated with glyphosate herbicides like Round-up. The purpose, besides providing weed control, is to kill the plant early for an easier and larger harvest. According to the USDA, 97-99% of durum and spring wheat is treated with these herbicides. Pesticide residues remaining on the wheat make their way into our digestive tract through the bread, pasta and other wheat products we eat. This can disrupt the functioning of beneficial bacteria in our guts and contribute to inflammatory and autoimmune disorders such as Celiac disease and certain cancers.

A fourth potential problem is the milling of wheat after removing the bran and wheat germ (containing valuable vitamins and micronutrients). The milling breaks down starch granules into a superfine flour which is digested too fast and absorbed into the blood instead of feeding our gut flora with its soluble fiber. Simply put, to increase shelf life, we take out important vitamins and nutrients and make a product that causes spikes in our blood sugar and inflammation in our gut.

A fifth problem with modern bread is the commercial baking process. Traditional bread making, which we practice at home, uses sourdough starter with naturally occurring bacteria and yeast from the surrounding air and requires hours for the dough to rise. Commercial bakers, however, often use fast-rising yeasts and "Vital Wheat Gluten" for faster rising of the dough. This denatured process is fast but does not give the yeast and bacteria enough time to digest some or all the high gluten content in the flour.

---

[19] https://www.totalresults.net/blog/?id=426

It is hard to know what exactly triggers gluten or wheat resistance in some people but if I suspected I had such a problem I would start by looking at the factors listed above, and follow the advice in this book about avoiding denatured grains and bread. I would also try to make my own sourdough bread at home, and add probiotic-rich fermented food and good fibers to my diet, before I completely eliminate gluten from my life. Our ancestors could not live with wheat and whole grains in their diet.

Antinutrients

ATI (wheat's natural pest-repellent) is one of the many natural compounds that plants, grains and beans contain or release to protect themselves against their hungry enemies. Although cooking and baking usually neutralizes some of these *antinutrient* compounds, they may still interfere with the metabolism of some minerals in some humans. Here are some examples of these antinutrients:

Lectins in some raw beans and nuts can impact absorption of iron, calcium, phosphorus and zinc in our body.

Phytic acid or phytates in corn, oat, pumpkin seeds, brown rice, and to a lesser extent in wheat and rye, can interfere with the absorption of calcium, magnesium iron and zinc in our body.

Oxalates found in spinach, dark leafy greens, rhubarb, kale, beans and nuts, tea and chocolate can also bind calcium in our body and may cause kidney stones.

Tannins in coffee and tea can bind iron and disrupt its metabolism in our body.

Glucosinolates in cabbage and cruciferous vegetables may bind with iodine and cause hypothyroidism.

It is best not to totally eliminate these foods from our diet because they are beneficial in many ways. Phytates for example can help with lowering cholesterol and blood sugar levels. They can also bind to excess calcium in our body and detoxify us.

Generally speaking, soaking, fermenting, sprouting and boiling grains and beans is known to reduce the levels of these antinutrients. Also eating foods with antinutrients in separate smaller portions and not together with other foods may prevent their disruptive effect on other nutrients and minerals. Another strategy is to consume antinutrients with some excess of nutrients. For example consuming phytate-rich food with yogurt products containing extra calcium, vitamins A and D could minimize its impact on our body's calcium balance and metabolism.

Some farmers and nutritionists blame modern farming practices such as monocultures and excessive application of phosphorus-based fertilizers for the high levels of phytates and antinutrients in modern food. Others blame infertile soils resulting from excessive plowing, tilling and run-off for Niacin (vitamin B3) deficiency in corn leading to diseases like Pellagra. That is why corn tortilla in Mexico is prepared using a technique called *nixtamalization* which includes cooking and steeping of maize in water mixed with food-grade powdered limestone. Others claim human bodies will adapt and adjust to these antinutrients over time especially if we eat fermented food that is symbiotic with our beneficial gut bacteria.

In my view, consuming large quantities of any single plant repeatedly, even good ones that are sprouted or fermented, could expose humans to abnormally high levels of antifeedant compounds. These are biochemicals used by nature to prevent mass elimination of any plant. Even the beneficial polyphenol compounds in berries, if consumed in large amounts, could trigger undesired immune responses in the human body.

Supplements

Purified, concentrated, isolated or synthetic forms of nutrients sold as supplements are generally not as "bioavailable" as their natural forms in raw food which are balanced with partnering cofactors such as enzymes, probiotics and minerals. Certain supplements, however, could be beneficial in cases of malnutrition and metabolic disorders, whether chronic or acute/seasonal. For example, low exposure to sunlight in cold and cloudy seasons could result in vitamin D deficiency and problems with calcium metabolism in people not consuming healthy cholesterol sources like pasture-raised raw milk and eggs. (Remember Vitamin D is synthesized by our skin from cholesterol type molecules and sunlight). Occasional use of good quality vitamin D supplements like cod liver oil from wild-caught fish, if not too old or oxidized, could mitigate vitamin D deficiency in some people.

Another example is good quality vitamin C, including the liposomal versions with rose hips or fermented types from organic fruits and vegetables, which is helpful in times of stress. But as with all supplements, it is not easy to independently evaluate the quality of the supplement or the accuracy of the assays and claims by the manufacturer.

There are countless supplements and herbal extracts on the market. Some of them seem to have legitimate therapeutic claims and some others seem to be of questionable quality or exaggerate their benefits. Those from natural organic sources or fermented from vegetables and fruits may offer better natural balance and bioavailability. High concentrations or super high doses of any purified or isolated nutrient, whether proteins, vitamins, fibers, or minerals are not natural and may cause serious metabolic disruptions in our body.

Detoxification

If we do not eat the right way, our body will be toxified and diseased. There are numerous *detoxification* protocols. The topic is beyond the scope of this book and I believe different "balancing" protocols (I prefer the word *balancing* because the goal of detoxification should be achieving metabolic balance) may be needed for different people depending on their imbalances and history. Because detox protocols use concentrated, extreme measures to correct our imbalances in a short time, they also have the potential of causing harm and further imbalances in our body if not done or formulated properly. Many detoxification (*detox* for short) protocols include:

* Chelating agents to extract heavy metals from the body. These include EDTA, zeolites, bentonite clays, activated charcoal, herbs and plant roots like dandelion roots, etc. Chelating agents can cause serious harm if not working properly.

* Heavy doses of herbs and vitamins like Vitamin C (supplements or vegetables) to fight and reverse oxidative cellular damages

* High fiber (prebiotic) and probiotic (fermented food or supplements) diets to populate good gut bacteria

* Low sugar, salt, seed oil, animal products (eggs, dairy, meat) to lower blood sugar, pressure and cholesterol

* Plenty of exercise and sweating (in sunlight or inside sauna or during exercise). Movement induces lymphatic flow and helps our immune system. Sweating will remove toxins from our body.

* Plenty of water (filtered), sunlight, sleep, relaxation, meditation (prayers) and peaceful (low stress) activities.

I believe these are important steps in detoxification, which are included in protocols like this one: https://www.fammed.wisc.edu/files/webfm-uploads/documents/outreach/im/handout_detoxplan.pdf. There are also other approaches to detoxification which may be simpler but may take longer, for example by switching to a lifestyle that allows you to follow the recommendations in this book about proper food, sleep and eating patterns.

In my studies, I have found the following ingredients as powerful natural agents to balance our metabolism in times of stress:

* For infections: Garlic, onions (including a compound called quercetin also found in apples and dark-skin grapes of less sweet, more fibrous old variety), thyme (activating mucosal immunity for respiratory infections), honey (from a trusted source, see my article on Substack about good honey from healthy bees). All chemical-free.

* For inflammations and immune system: Turmeric, black seed oil, Cod liver oil (Vitamin D), Vitamin C in Vegetables (chemical-free pepper, lemon, tomatoes potatoes, etc.), Fermented foods (kefir from whole raw pasture-raised milk, chemical-free sauerkraut)

* For good fiber, digestive clean up (soluble/insoluble fiber): Barley (in soup or as a meal or bread), Oatmeal (with honey and milk), potato (all chemical-free), heirloom apples (not overly sweet or soft)

* For micronutrients: Colorful fruits like berries, tomatoes, carrots (all chemical-free)

* Movement (walking, gardening or farming) under sunshine and adjusting our circadian biorhythm (meal and sleep times) with sunrise and sunset

* Fasting or Restricted Eating: Helpful with detoxification if the body is not fighting with acute or serious diseases that drain its energy

* Deep slow breathing and conscious control over your breath throughout the day (exhalation of at least 8 seconds)

Ancient Asian physiology and medicine, focusing on the entire body as a whole system, used the body's own "purging" mechanisms for detoxification. In times of serious toxicity, metabolic disorders, and disease they recommended the following (Caution: If self-administered excessively, regularly or improperly, some of these purging methods can cause more harm than good):

* Laxatives and Enema therapy: To expel toxins from the guts, castor oil has been used as a natural laxative. Enema therapy has also been practiced for colon cleansing and general detoxification, using herbs or coffee. In recent years, Dr. Max Gerson suggested coffee enema for the treatment of degenerative diseases such as skin tuberculosis, diabetes, and cancer.

* Emetics to Induce Vomiting: Completely clearing stomach of its contents on an occasional basis using herbs like hyssop (the mint family) or warm 5% saline on empty stomach, was used historically to detoxify people with poor digestion, high phlegm, slow metabolism (especially in winter months), heavy weight or diets high in high fat. In traditional Chinese medicine vomiting was also used to cleanse the liver and spleen due to their connection to the stomach in the digestive system (bile processing). Voluntary- induced vomiting is also a yogic cleansing technique which is believed to strengthen respiratory muscles and enhance air flow in our lungs (for deep breathing). Vomiting also resembles the valsalva maneuver (increasing our intrathoracic pressure which happens when we blow up a balloon, strain during defecation, or play the saxophone) which stimulates our Vagus nerve and relaxation (parasympathetic), healing mode.

* Bloodletting by phlebotomy, cupping or leeches has been used in ancient and alternative medicine to promote

healing, remove toxins, relieve pain, and restore the body's energy flow. In Ayurvedic therapies, bloodletting is believed to detoxify the body as happens regularly during menstruation for women. Greek physician Galen advocated bloodletting to treat seriously infected patients. In 18th century Europe, bloodletting was done by barbers! Occasional blood loss is shown to mitigate erythrocytosis (too much hemoglobin, thick blood) and infectious iron overload.

* Anointment and Oil Rubbing: Practiced in ancient times with unrefined virgin oils (olive, black seed, sesame, or essential oils like clove, thyme or Frankincense) for healing and religious consecration. In both animals and plants, the function of the surface (skin) sebaceous oil with acidic pH is to keep toxins and harmful bacteria outside and keep valuable nutrients and fluids within. Following infections and sweating, anointing with oil may be a good step to reduce sweating, when used in conjunction with bathing because it closes pores. Certain essential oils like clove, thyme, Eucalyptus, lemongrass, or Frankincense have antibacterial and antifungal properties. In some ancient detoxification practices, *navel therapy* included rubbing warm virgin oils such as black seed, almond, coconut, sesame or essential oils (chemical-free) to the navel (belly button) before bed time to boost immune system, stimulate the vagus nerve (relaxation) and reduce pains and inflammations.

* Diuretics and Sweating: Our body naturally sweats in times of serious infection to rid itself of toxins and excess heat. Urination is also a pathway for water-soluble toxins to leave our body. Some traditional detoxification protocols induced extra urination by the use of natural diuretics like asparagus, parsley, celery. Extra sweating can also be induced (in non-feverish patients) by exposure to sunlight and sauna.

* Gandhi's Approach to Detoxification: The leader of India's independence, Mohandas Gandhi was also a well-read sage, a vegetarian and a practitioner of ancient detoxification protocols, and those promoted in Adolf Just's *Return To Nature* and Louis Kuhne's *Neo Naturopathy: The New Science of Healing.* Gandhi believed humans should eat sparingly, and fast and pray regularly. He experimented with hydrotherapy and mud therapy, which helped with his occasional headaches and constipation. In mud therapy, he applied a mud poultice made from clean red earth (clay powder, heated and sterilized, not from sprayed or fertilized soil) to his head or abdomen. Today, some detox protocols also use pure bentonite (Montmorillonite) clay powders or activated charcoal as topical treatments to remove toxins or cleanse the skin.

Concluding Epilogue

Remember, you have access to subsidized or free "medicine" *after* you get sick, but when it comes to good "food" to *prevent* disease, you are on your own[20]! Many of the foods we eat today ravage our guts, which (as explained) are called our "second brain" because they are innervated by the second largest neural network in our body (after our brain), including the all-important vagus nerve, and host the largest bacterial colony in our body responsible for making serotonin, the body's important modulator of the immune system, mood, digestion and metabolic balance.

Good gut-healthy food ingredients are produced (cultivated) in smaller quantities and with care, so they are not that profitable as a business. Families who run "small chemical-free" farms like ours that use regenerative methods *not* exploiting illegal labor or big expensive tractors (bought on bank loans), are hard-pressed to make more than $20 an hour for their

---

[20] Available subsidies often go to large-scale conventional (spraying) farms

labor. So if you make more than $20 an hour, buying locally fresh vegetables, grains and fruits from these types of farms is the best investment you can make in your health because you are basically hiring someone else and their land to grow top quality food for you at less than your own hourly income. If you make less than $20 an hour, it is economically and metabolically wise to find ways to free up your time and some land to grow "some" of your own vegetables and easy sources of starch, vitamins and micronutrients like potatoes.

If you have children and a backyard, you can easily teach your family how to grow potatoes without any chemicals (pesticides) and just by using some hay or (unsprayed) grass mulch. Start with good heirloom type (chemical-free) potato seeds. You can learn growing potatoes in old books by The Rodale Press or other homesteading or vegetable gardening books. Children like harvesting potatoes because they dig and find gold-looking potatoes as reward for their hard work and learn how to feed themselves. You can get neighbors' children to help with seeding and harvesting too. You can harvest 300 pounds from a 20 ft by 40 ft plot, which is enough healthy starch for a family of 4 throughout the year if stored in a cool and dark (and not too dry) place. I wrote in Substack about potato's nutritional facts and interesting history. Potatoes are great foods in times of crisis because they store well and are very nutritious.

Remember, your health, i.e., your body functions and vitality (energy levels without medicine, sugar, coffee, stimulants), is your indicator of how healthy your food is. If you experience any of the 4 S's of metabolic disorder, namely dysfunctions in sleep, stool (one bowel movement a day, not too runny or hard), sense of smell and sexual/reproductive health, you need to find the time and or money to eat the right way.

Like all other good things in life, researching, finding, growing and preparing good food takes *time.* All blessings of life also need people who *care.* Consider yourself blessed if you have farmers around you who *care* about the vegetables they grow, the soil they grow it in, the chickens they raise for eggs, etc. Buy from them and encourage others to buy from them too. There are not many small chemical-free farms left any more. If you have to buy some of your food ingredients from commercial quality, mass- produced food suppliers, be picky and find the level of denaturation by researching the sources and practices used to grow it. Be particularly vigilant on food from animal sources (meat, eggs, dairy).

About a century ago, a large number of Americans grew food for themselves and their neighboring towns. The Pennsylvania Triennial Farm Census in 1927 shows that many rural households had apple, pear and peach trees, chickens, cows, fields of potato, wheat, oats and corn. Today, food, medicine and supplements are big *global* (non-local, mass-produced) profitable businesses. People no longer personally know the farmer producing milk, vegetables and eggs for them. So everyone must be a wise supermarket customer. There is a lot of *misinformation* out there. Some large food businesses also own divisions that make tobacco (cigarettes) and alcohol. The manufacturer of glyphosate-based herbicides (used in farms), suspected to cause non-Hodgkin's lymphoma (cancer), also makes money by developing anti-cancer drugs!

When it comes to eating healthy, nothing beats setting aside "as much time as needed" to grow your own or find fresh, unadulterated and seasonal ingredients, to cook and make your own meals fresh at home from these ingredients, and to constantly learn and educate yourself and others about healthy food. Please help folks like me spread the word. A sick society is a weak society, and easier to control and manipulate than a healthy one.

Made in the USA
Columbia, SC
13 September 2024

41599552R00064